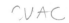

The Sweet Bloods of Eeyou Istchee

Stories of Diabetes and the James Bay Cree
Second Edition

Stories by James Bay Cree Storytellers

Written by Ruth DyckFehderau

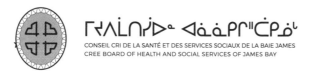

ᒥᔅᐃᓈᐱᔨᐆᐤ ᐊᓈᓈᐱᒋᐦᒡᐸᑯ�

CONSEIL CRI DE LA SANTÉ ET DES SERVICES SOCIAUX DE LA BAIE JAMES
CREE BOARD OF HEALTH AND SOCIAL SERVICES OF JAMES BAY

Funding for this publication was provided in part by Health Canada. The opinions expressed in this publication are those of the story-tellers and do not necessarily reflect the official views of Health Canada or of Cree Board of Health and Social Services of James Bay.

Some names and details in this book have been changed for the purpose of protecting identities. Any similarities between these changed names or details and real persons, living or dead, is not intended.

First edition, 2017. Second edition, 2020.
Printed and bound in Canada by Houghton Boston Printers, Saskatoon, Saskatchewan.
Distributed by Wilfrid Laurier University Press: wlupress.wlu.ca

Set in Verdana font, chosen for its readability. Printed on paper that is Forest Stewardship Council-certified with post-consumer recycled fibres, and that is acid- and chlorine-free.

Cover design by Cameron Mosimann of Edmonton, Alberta.
Photograph of Mistissini burnt forest (reversed) taken by David DyckFehderau.
Map adapted from official Cree Board of Health and Social Services of James Bay map.

Copyright © 2020 Cree Board of Health and Social Services of James Bay
Published by Cree Board of Health and Social Services of James Bay
Contact: Paul Linton, 168 Main St, Mistissini, QC. G0W 1C0.
418.923.3355

sweetbloods.org | creehealth.org

Includes bibliographical references.
ISBN 978-0-9730542-4-8 (softcover)
First edition available in audiobook format.

Library and Archives Canada Cataloguing in Publication

Title: The sweet bloods of Eeyou Istchee : stories of diabetes and the James Bay Cree / stories by James Bay Cree storytellers ; written by Ruth DyckFehderau.
Names: DyckFehderau, Ruth, author. | Cree Board of Health and Social Services of James Bay, publisher.
Description: Second edition. | Includes bibliographical references.
Identifiers: Canadiana 20200233602 | ISBN 9780973054248 (softcover)
Subjects: LCSH: Diabetes—Québec (Province)—Nord-du-Québec. | LCSH: Diabetics—Québec (Province)—Nord-du-Québec—Biography. | LCSH: Cree Indians—Health and hygiene—Québec (Province)—Nord-du-Québec.
Classification: LCC RA645.D5 D93 2020 | DDC 362.1964/62009714115—dc23

The Sweet Bloods of Eeyou Istchee

Stories of Diabetes and the James Bay Cree: Second Edition

STORYTELLERS

Rose Swallow
Simon Etapp
Varley Mianscum
Mary Niquanicappo
Kimberly Coon
Martha Sheshamush
Leonard House
Jennifer Gloria Lowpez*
Jennifer Susan Annistin*
Jack Otter
Caroline Neeposh
Anja Diamond*
Joey Blacksmith
Freddie Wapachee

Maggie Happyjack
Annette Spencer
Sandra Judith Bulluck*
Victor Gilpin
James Allan Jonah
Emily Wesley
Elizabeth Bell Tayler*
Christopher Merriman
Raquel Emmeline Welsch*
Lillian Martinhunter
Jonathan Linton
Angela Etapp
Coco Simone Chanelle*

*Names have been changed

ALL STORIES WRITTEN BY Ruth DyckFehderau

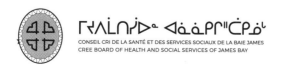

ᒥᐛᓕᐣᔨᐅᓐ ᐊᓐᓇᐱᕐᐦᑕᕐᓐᑯᓯᐤ

CONSEIL CRI DE LA SANTÉ ET DES SERVICES SOCIAUX DE LA BAIE JAMES
CREE BOARD OF HEALTH AND SOCIAL SERVICES OF JAMES BAY

*For the storytellers
of Eeyou Istchee*

Contents

Eeyou Istchee

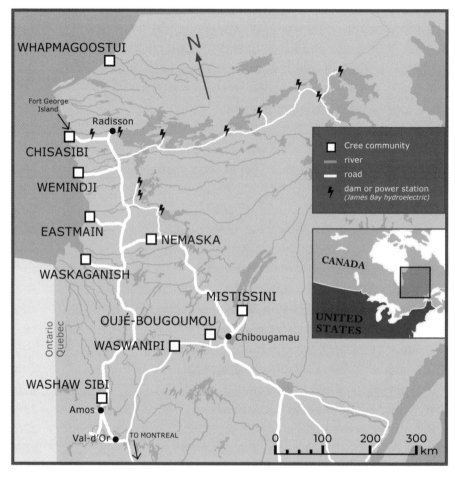

WHAPMAGOOSTUI

Fort George Island

Radisson

CHISASIBI

WEMINDJI

EASTMAIN

NEMASKA

WASKAGANISH

MISTISSINI

OUJÉ-BOUGOUMOU

Chibougamau

WASWANIPI

Ontario
Quebec

WASHAW SIBI

Amos

Val-d'Or

TO MONTREAL

Cree community
river
road
dam or power station
(James Bay hydroelectric)

CANADA

UNITED STATES

0   100   200   300
km

Some Notes About This Book

THIS is a book of stories told by James Bay Cree of Northern Québec—or, the Eeyou (Cree of the Interior) and Eenou (Cree of the Eastern James Bay Coast) who live on the territory of Eeyou Istchee—for Cree and other Indigenous peoples of Canada.

The James Bay Cree of Northern Québec, at time of writing, are made up of ten (out of 6341[1]) distinct First Nations communities[2] of Canada. They include the Whapmagoostui First Nation, the Cree Nation of Chisasibi, the Cree Nation of Wemindji, the Cree Nation of Eastmain, Waskaganish First Nation, the Cree Nation of Washaw Sibi, Nemaska First Nation, the Cree First Nation of Waswanipi, the Cree Nation of Mistissini, and Ouجé-Bougoumou Cree Nation. Their traditional land region, Eeyou Istchee, is roughly 450,000 square kilometres.[3] They use the region in its entirety, and they have lived there for at least 5500 to 8000 years, depending on the source.[4]

1. "Description of the AFN." *Assembly of First Nations.* AFN. Web. 05 Mar 2016.
2. The First Nations are one of three main Indigenous groups in Canada. The other two are the Inuit and the Métis.
3. Cree Nations of Eeyou Istchee. "The Cree Vision of Plan Nord" *Grand Council of the Crees (Eeyou Istchee): Publications and Resources.* (February 2011):16. Web. 25 Feb 2016.
4. According to David Denton, archaeologist with the Cree Nation Government, the Aanischaaukamikw Cree Cultural Institute in Ouجé-Bougoumou holds Cree objects that have been carbon-14 dated to 5500 years of age, and local Cree cultural experts speak in casual conversation of history and objects going back more than 8000 years. By comparison, the Egyptian pyramids are roughly 4500 years old.

This book includes stories from nine of the ten communities. At time of writing, Washaw Sibi, the tenth community, was still in the process of being established as a distinct First Nation community. It is mentioned in the stories, but none of the storytellers here call it their home.

Eeyou Istchee has a disproportionately high prevalence of diabetes. In some communities, fully one-third of the adults have been diagnosed with type 2 or gestational diabetes and more remain undiagnosed. To address this prevalence and to demystify the disease, the Cree Board of Health and Social Services of James Bay (CBHSSJB) has, in recent decades, launched a number of solutions.[5] This book is one of them. Under the *Aboriginal Diabetes Initiative,*[6] these stories have been collected with goals of nurturing open and informed discussion, of correcting misinformation about the disease, of encouraging people living with diabetes, and of sharing ways that Eeyou and Eenou cope (or don't cope), thrive (or don't thrive), with diabetes.

The book was envisioned as a type of Talking Circle. Traditionally, the Cree come together in Talking Circles to tell and hear stories or to speak and listen on a subject. The Circles assume, first, that all the parts of life and history that make up a human being or a human-being story cannot be separated from one another, that health and wellness or disease and sickness might be as much about a spiritual or emotional or intellectual part of a person as they are about her or his physical being; second, the

5. For instance, CBHSSJB trained local Community Health Representatives (CHRs) to provide a crossing point between Cree with diabetes and physicians, and to speak to people about diabetes in their own language. Additionally, CBHSSJB launched a documentary called *Sweet Blood: Live Well with Diabetes (Dir. Shirley Cheechoo, 2009),* a film that encourages making gradual changes in diet and exercise to manage diabetes. The film also notes that some Cree with type 2 diabetes who have returned to a traditional diet of mainly wild game and to a traditional active life have seen a partial or full reversal of symptoms. The title of this book is taken from the *Sweet Blood* documentary.
6. The *Aboriginal Diabetes Initiative* is an initiative funded by the federal government of Canada aimed at reducing type 2 diabetes in Indigenous communities. The initiative focuses on preventing diabetes through culturally relevant means and approaches.

circles assume that the act of storytelling is a healing act both for the individual and for the community; and third, they assume that individual healing cannot be separated from community healing. In this case, the vast distances between communities of Eeyou Istchee prevented the 27 storytellers from gathering in the same room as they would in a traditional Talking Circle, but the stories are gathered here to do the work that Talking Circles do: to share, to solve problems and help make community decisions, to process and pass on information, and to heal.

My personal motivation as the writer of the stories was much simpler: I tried to listen carefully to each storyteller, and then, as best I could, to put onto the page her or his story and words along with the voice and emotions that circled the room during storytelling. Put another way, my goal was above all to honour the storytellers and their stories.

In November of 2012, I was living in Mistissini, Eeyou Istchee, working on a novel, when I was hired by CBHSSJB to write the stories in this storybook project.

We started the project with a pilot story. One of the storytellers in this book told me his story, and I wrote it up in different ways. The CBHSSJB Assistant Director of Public Health for Chishaayiyuu (adults) and I agreed that the short story format, rather than news journalism or word-for-word interviews, was the format most suited to the project. The story approach resonated with the storytellers as well.

At this point in the project, Community Health Representatives (CHRs) in each community looked at their lists of individuals with diabetes and chose a few whom they thought might enjoy participating in the project, or whose stories they thought especially valuable to a collection such as this one. The choices made by the CHRs were not directed in any way, and we made no attempt to get a representative cross-section of demographic profiles. The CHRs contacted the individuals they had chosen, 28 in total, and set up meetings. People participated if they wanted to do so.

I flew to each community then, and sat down in a quiet room with each of the individual storytellers. I pressed play on the recording devices, and I listened as carefully as I could to whatever the storytellers wanted to tell me. From time to time, I asked questions for clarification or chatted on a topic that had come up, but the conversations took their natural course and I tried not to push them in one direction or another. I did not enter these conversations with a specific set of interview questions as a conventional researcher might do. In fact, I didn't approach these conversations as interviews at all.

After returning to my home, I wrote up the individual conversations into drafts of short stories. I relied on the claims of the storytellers and aimed to write the stories in a way that resonated with the teller and the teller's account. Once the drafts were completed, I travelled back to each community again and went through the stories with the individual storytellers. The storytellers corrected errors I had made, and each one confirmed that her or his story said what s/he wanted it to say. I trusted their accounts and edits absolutely and did no further fact-checking myself. At this point, some of the storytellers requested anonymity, and one storyteller withdrew from the project altogether for personal reasons. I made any and all changes the storytellers requested, and then I destroyed all original recordings and drafts and notes (which sometimes contained personal matters that had come up in conversation and that storytellers did not wish to include in the final product). The finished pieces in this collection, approved by the storytellers, are all that remains.

Because I am not Cree (nor Indigenous at all), because I have only studied and not experienced Cree history, and because I do not speak the Cree language (thereby forcing most of the storytellers to recount their stories in a language other than their first), there are undoubtedly errors in this text. Further, storytelling is a dynamic activity and the stories here reflect only what the storytellers were comfortable sharing with me on the days we met. We attempted to address some of the shortcomings by having the storytellers check and re-check their own stories. But certainly the storytellers' accounts contained subtleties and nuances that I simply did not have the ability to hear or understand and was consequently unable to transfer to the page.

It is no small thing to enter a quiet room and tell your story in detail to a stranger in a language other than your own. Each person who did it here stated, without being prompted, that s/he was doing it to help other people. My unending gratitude goes to the storytellers in this volume for their generosity of time and spirit and for the willingness to share their stories.

Ruth DyckFehderau (Writer)

1

The Story of Rose Swallow of Chisasibi

WHEN Rose was a young girl, not yet in school, she and her grandfather swaddled against the cold bay wind and took the dog-sled over Hudson Bay and up La Grande River to check the fishnets. Rose perched up on the sled, the sun glinted off snowdrifts around her, the frenzied huskies kicked up snow in front of her, and her grandfather ran alongside the sled. Sometimes he jumped on for a minute or two of rest.

"Look," he said then, "you can see how smart the dogs are. They know where the ice is thin and they avoid it. We can go to my river nets, where the water runs faster and the ice is more danger-ous, only because of them."

He didn't want to tire the huskies with his extra weight, though, and soon hopped off the sled again to lope along beside.

When they reached a fishnet, Rose climbed down from the sled and the dogs rested while her grandfather, after all that running, heaved up the catch. The net was so heavy with ice and water and fish that his body leaned back on an angle and his arms and legs strained with the weight of it. He untangled the fish from the net, bashed them on the ice to kill them quickly, bundled them and lashed the bundle to the sled. Rose climbed back on top of the load, and they were off again, on to the next net, grandfather running beside.

Back at the cabin at the end of the day, her grandfather cooked up a big meal with bones and meat and rice for the dogs.

"You must feed dogs well," he said. "Every day, twice a day, and not only on the days they pull the sled. Never be cruel to a dog; you have to respect each one."

Only after the dogs were fed did he sit down himself and rest.

In the summers, when fish were more plentiful, Rose helped her grandmother build a drying rack from saplings and sinew. They straddled it across a damp-wood fire and together they draped fish over the rack to smoke until they were well-preserved. They wrapped the fish up in a cloth from a flour sack and loaded the bundles into sacks. Then they carted the sacks on their backs to her grand-mother's cache, a storage area 15 minutes away that she had dug out underground and lined with moss for insulation. They placed the fish bundles inside the moss where they would stay cool and piled on top the heaviest rocks they could find so the wolves couldn't get at them.

The big and small game—moose and caribou and grouse and rabbit—was all hunted on foot, or caught in snares and traps that her grandparents would walk to every week. Over long afternoons, Rose's grandmother would slow-cook the game into stews and float soft dumplings in the dark gravies. The flour had been purchased in town and sometimes, when there was enough of it, she made bannock to sop up the juices.

Berry-picking time came around August, when the blueberries were a deep navy and had sweetened in the sun. Rose and her grand-parents walked out in the afternoons and picked all they could find. Her grandmother boiled some berries into jams or folded them into cakes, and the rest she dried and preserved in a cotton bag where they wouldn't mould. And with the fish and the berries and other hunted meats, they had food in the long winter months.

Some years, the years of starving, were bad. Even with the fishing and the hunting and the berry-picking, there wasn't enough food. Then Rose's grandfather would go out to the islands in the bay. There was a lichen that grew there; it was something like a black moss and something like lettuce. You could boil it, if you had to, and eat it. It would get you through the bad times.

It was an athletic life, living on the land. You were always moving, just to be able to eat. Always doing something. No one in the area had heard of diabetes then.

The year after the dogsled rides to the fishnets, Rose sat in the residential school dining room contemplating something on her plate. The teachers called it "broccoli" and Rose was supposed to eat it—but it didn't look like food. She was being watched, though: if she didn't clean her plate she would be punished and either starved or beaten until she couldn't get out of bed. And so she closed her eyes, tried to think about the parts of her school day that she enjoyed—like French class and baking class and handicrafts—and she stabbed her fork into that vile broccoli stem and willed her mouth to open. When she closed it, bitter juices squirted across her tongue and in seconds the broccoli became a revolting mush. All around her in the dining room, Cree kids were gagging and vomiting at the strange food. This had to be worse than that black lichen her grandparents had eaten in the starving times. But Rose forced it down and avoided a beating. *When I grow up*, she thought, *I will have kids. And I will never force them to eat broccoli.* In those years, there was still no talk of diabetes.

In the late '60s, Rose walked into the bathroom of her high school in Rouyn-Noranda. Another student was there: a girl who had hiked up her skirt, propped her leg up on the big round water fountain—and was sliding a needle into the flesh of her thigh. *A heroin addict,* thought Rose, *right here, in my high school!* Rose washed her hands at the fountain and returned to class without saying anything to the girl. A few years later, though, in Biology class, the girl came to mind again. The teacher talked about the pancreas and a disease called diabetes which was treated with injections of insulin. That needle girl had been injecting not heroin but insulin, Rose realized, and without it she would have died. She was the first person with diabetes that Rose ever saw.

Rose finished her schooling and found work at the Chisasibi Hudson's Bay Store. It was the '70s, a time of big changes. Hunters and fishermen used snowmobiles for their work and no longer ran alongside dog-pulled sleds. Many of the dogs were neither respected nor looked after. Locals didn't walk to the grocery store anymore; they drove for even the smallest errand and trucks and cars crowded the narrow streets. For the first time, the store began to stock televisions. People bought them up so quickly the store couldn't keep them stocked. CBC was the only channel in those days, and it was on for just an hour a day—but when that hour came, people all around town stopped whatever they were doing to go to their living room or the living room of someone who had a TV. And they sat immobile for an entire hour looking at the screen and watching the news.

A Métis lady, about 50 years old, worked with Rose at the store in those days, and she was thirsty. She stuck some price tickets on a stack of boxes, then hustled over to the water fountain, gulped a whole cup of water, and came back to work. One minute later, she needed to drink again. She drank and drank, all day long, but couldn't quench her thirst. Rose could see the desperation on her face, as if she would die of thirst even after having so much water, and it was something terrible. Another lady working there saw all this, and noticed too that the thirsty lady's vision had gotten much worse in a few weeks. She gently told the thirsty lady to go to the doctor—she had heard about an illness that made people thirsty and affected their eyesight. Maybe there was some medicine. A few days later, the thirsty lady was back at work with an enormous glass-and-metal syringe. She stabbed the needle into a bottle of insulin, pulled back to fill the syringe, and injected it into her flesh every single day. She would have to do this, she said, for the rest of her life. Sometimes the insulin wouldn't be enough; she would feel shaky and would run to the coffee tray and pop a sugar cube into her mouth. She was the second person with diabetes that Rose ever met.

Then, suddenly, talk of diabetes was everywhere in the community. Rose's friends and neighbours, several elders, even her family had diabetes. One by one, Rose's seven sisters were diagnosed, and one of them even had two miscarriages as a result of the disease. In 1991, Rose began working as a Community Health Representative (CHR) for the Cree Board of Health and Social Services of James Bay. Twenty years had passed since she had met the thirsty lady and thirty years since she had seen the girl with the needle in high school, and now Rose worked every day with people with diabetes. More people were being newly diagnosed every month—and almost every one of them was surprised.

"That can't be right," they would say to her. "I never eat sweets. It can't be diabetes."

Rose would explain to each person, in the Cree language that the doctors and nurses couldn't speak, that the flour in dumplings and bannock might not taste sweet, but it was a kind of sugar nevertheless.

"But," they would say, "our grandparents ate bannock and dumplings and they didn't have diabetes."

"Yes," Rose would answer, "they ate bannock and dumplings. But think of all the exercise they did that we don't do. Think of all the ways our lives are different from theirs."

She began talking about diabetes on the radio and in schools, teaching people not to have both rice and potatoes in the same meal because both are a kind of sugar, teaching that a long walk would lower blood sugar for up to two days, teaching that alcohol could be dense with sugar even if it didn't taste sweet, teaching that stress aggravated the disease. And still, there were so many new diagnoses of diabetes and other chronic illnesses that Rose couldn't do all the work herself and the Cree Board of Health had to hire another CHR for Chisasibi just to meet the demand.

And then another.

And then another.

From time to time, Rose used the glucose-testing kits to screen herself. She didn't have diabetes symptoms, but it ran in her family and there was quite a bit of stress in her home in those days, before her husband stopped drinking. So many people in the community were getting sick. For years her test results were fine but Rose continued self-screening. For years, she brought test kits home from work and tested her husband and all her kids. She even did what she had vowed never to do: she made her children eat broccoli—but without even once using the extreme residential school methods.

One day, in '97, her self-screening showed a new result: pre-diabetes, a warning sign that diabetes was not far away. Rose began to take medication and became still more diligent about exercise and careful eating. Then, on a sunny day in spring 2002, she went to the bathroom at work and remembered, as she zipped up her pants, that she had been to the bathroom just ten minutes earlier—and ten minutes before that. She could already feel she would need the toilet in a few minutes again. She crossed the office to the cupboard with the test kits. She pricked her finger with the lancet, wiped the blood on the strip, and inserted it into the reader. The number in the glucose reader was too high. Rose Swallow, like the needle girl in high school and the thirsty lady from the Hudson's Bay Store, like every one of her sisters, had diabetes.

She sucked in a deep breath and let it out. And then she ran back to the bathroom.

Rose is still a CHR in Chisasibi, along with four other CHRs. She's in charge of the diabetes portfolio and spends most of her work time teaching people, in their own language, how to manage the disease. By now, every Chisasibi family is directly affected by diabetes and the newly diagnosed are getting younger and younger. Rose organizes healthy-food tastings. Vegetables and fruits are so expensive in the North that people don't want to spend money on new ones they might not like, so Rose finds ways to let them taste new foods without having to pay all that money. She also organizes Leave-Your-Vehicle-At-Home days for people to try exercising as a way of getting to work, as their grandparents once did. And she encourages people to try the fitness centre, even if it is a little intimidating at first. Chisasibi is seeing big changes again: people are exercising more, walking outside along the highway or the river in the long summer evenings, or snowshoeing across the open spaces in winter. So far, though, Rose hasn't seen anyone running alongside a dog team.

Like all the people she teaches, Rose has to work at her own diabetes every day. She takes her pills and tests her blood sugar. She experiments with vegetables and cooks with whole grains and high fibre. She has to be especially careful about stress— it's the one thing that drives up her blood sugar levels very quickly. Sometimes calming down is as easy as taking a few deep breaths or reading a good book. Years ago, her husband's drinking was what drove up her anxiety, but he hasn't had a drink in years. These days, Rose worries for her kids and grandkids and also looks after some of her grandkids on the days they're neglected. It gets to be a lot of work and anxiety for someone no longer young enough to sit on her grandfather's dogsled.

Then her husband says, "Oh Rosie. I can see on your face—it's time to go for a walk."

And they tie on their boots and swaddle the grandkids against the cold and head out for a long walk by the highway where the sun glints off the snowdrifts and the grandkids kick up snow around them.

Stories We Heard Along the Way: Visitors

A while back, not too long after the town of Fort George was relocated to Chisasibi, the Russian government became gravely concerned over something they saw on satellite photos: structures in Chisasibi looked suspiciously like hiding places for secret missiles! They sent Russian experts to Ottawa to investigate. The Ottawa government people welcomed them and assured the Russians that the James Bay Cree were too busy with other things to bother about missiles and they should visit the town and see for themselves. And so the Russians paid Chisasibi a visit and saw that those "missile structures" were actually the homes and buildings that had been moved from the island and arranged in circles. And then they feasted on traditional foods with the local people, and went back home to Russia.

•

In 2005, a group of ten hunting tourists came to Northern Québec from France and shot a black bear. The Indigenous people of Québec have known for a long time that bear meat, fresh or frozen, must be cooked thoroughly before eating because it sometimes contains a parasite (*trichinella*) that can make people very sick, and this parasite even survives freezing. The French hunting tourists didn't take this cooking advice, though, and some of them ate the meat rare and others even tasted it raw. Two of them liked it so much that they smuggled pieces of bear meat back to France in their suitcases to share with friends and families. A week or two later, hospitals in France began seeing people who were very sick with *trichinellosis*, the infection that results from eating meat with the *trichinella* parasite in it—and all of them had eaten undercooked meat from the same bear. In total, about 25 people ate meat from the northern bear and most of them got very sick.

•

Some tropical cockroaches wanted to see the world and hitched a ride to Mistissini in a box of bananas. When they arrived, the cockroaches found that they liked Mistissini with its lovely view of the lake and, like the European colonizers who came hundreds of years earlier, decided to stay and take over. The box they had travelled in was good-sized, and it ended up in the basement of a house where their population grew and grew. Those cockroaches liked it so much that they didn't want to leave, even after they had taken over the house and outstayed their welcome. After a while, the house had so many cockroaches in it that the people had to move out and Public Health and Safety burned it down. Tropical cockroach tourism has since slowed considerably.

2

The Story of Maggie Happyjack and Simon Etapp of Waswanipi

THIS is a story about two people, Maggie and Simon, from the small town of Waswanipi, Québec. When the humidity is high and the sun is up, Maggie and Simon feel it in their ears, in the places where their eardrums once broke and healed, and they know that the weather lady will say there's a low-pressure system moving over James Bay tonight, it's time to settle in for some weather.

Simon is older than Maggie, so this story starts with him. He was born in the bush outside of Mistissini with a heart condition. The doctors said he'd outgrow it, and eventually he did, but when he was a child it was quite severe and his parents or other people looking after him would sometimes find him on the ground, unconscious, and they'd know his heart was acting up again. The heart condition was so bad that Simon's father thought he wouldn't live to adulthood. Even so, the Indian Affairs people sent Simon from his home away to Shingwauk Residential School in Sault Ste. Marie when he was very young. So young he couldn't yet tie his shoes. So young that the school sent him back home, saying he was too young even for them. (He wouldn't remember that part later;

someone else told him about it.) Unfortunately, Indian Affairs just sent him right back to the school.

For a boy so young, Shingwauk was a scary place. The building seemed huge to Simon. Along with the other young boys, he slept in a long dorm room with many beds and tall windows. The older kids slept upstairs. There was a scary counsellor, a lady, who was old and strict and fond of hitting kids with a stick, and there was a metal fire escape that didn't quite reach the ground and scared little kids like Simon. What made it worse was that both of Simon's parents were sick. His mom was in the hospital and the doctor had ordered shoulder surgery for his dad. Away from people who loved him—people who were sick—and in a place where he was often afraid, Simon began to worry that he might never see his parents again.

One day, Simon and his friends were playing out in the snow, sliding down the hill. His sled crossed a trail and got too close to a branch and Simon cut his cheek. He left his friends and went to the Infirmary, where the nurse bandaged his face and sent him to dorm to rest. There, in his dorm room at Shingwauk, he passed out onto his bed.

Anyone looking on would have seen Simon collapse, unconscious again, his heart condition acting up, all in a day's routine. But for Simon this time was different. His heart came to a full stop. His spirit left his body and floated up around the lightbulb in the ceiling and then through the ceiling, and then through the roof, and then above the clouds. He could see everything below getting smaller and smaller as he kept going up. Waiting for him, above the clouds, was an angel, bright and white with arms open to receive him. The angel looked at Simon kindly, and then sent him back down, back down through the clouds, through the roof, through the ceiling, onto the bed, and back into his body.

Simon sat up in his bed. A tray of food was waiting for him. He didn't know who had brought it, but he picked up a fork and began to eat.

He didn't tell anyone about that experience, not even his parents, for about fifty-five years.

Shingwauk was no picnic, but after a few years Indian Affairs sent Simon to the Mohawk Institute Residential School in Brantford—and for Simon that was worse. All the Native kids knew, Brantford was *bad.* It was one of the oldest Anglican Residential Schools in Canada and the people there had been practising how to hurt children for so long that they had gotten pretty good at it. They were so good at it that many of the kids who went to Brantford died while they were there, and more never made it home again. Mohawk kids had been sent to Brantford since the 1820s, but the Cree had been lucky to mostly avoid it for over a hundred years. Simon and his brother and two sisters were among the first unfortunate Cree to attend the place.

This is the part of the story where Maggie comes in. She was also from James Bay, from the community of Waswanipi. She didn't actually meet Simon properly until years later, but they were both Cree kids in the hell that was the Mush Hole. The good part was that they both survived. The bad part was everything else.

When they arrived, the first thing that happened was that girls and boys were separated. Maggie had come with her brother, (in later years, a second brother would join them), but he was put into a different dorm and she could have no contact with him at all. Every now and then, the single-file line-up of girls was in the yard at the same time as the single-file line-up of boys, and then she could at least lay her eyes on him, know he was still there, and move her fingers in a silent wave. As for Simon, if Maggie had noticed him in one of those line-ups, it would have been too risky to let him know.

The second thing that happened after they arrived was a haircut: Maggie got the same haircut as every other girl, and her brother and Simon and all the other boys had their heads shaved bald. At that time, when Maggie was still healthy from a summer at home where she had had plenty to eat, a nurse would mark down her height and weight and give her a quick look-over. Maggie usually wouldn't see a nurse again, or have anyone do anything for her health at all, until she went home in spring to the people who loved her—but by then she was pounds lighter and nearly starved.

People called Brantford Mohawk Institute the Mush Hole because the food was so bad. Through the crack in the door, Maggie could see the teachers eating good meals, she could smell roast beef and potatoes and green beans in butter, but she and the other kids were made to eat porridge that had long ago been overrun with worms. Most of the worms were dead, boiled with the porridge, but sometimes a hardy one had survived and it still wiggled a bit, making the porridge surface heave. When the food wasn't worm-infested, it was too strange to eat. Even if it was something they could recognize, say potatoes or corn, it would be cooked down, mixed with other things, and creamed into a slop that could hardly be swallowed. Or animal parts they knew shouldn't be eaten—like pig skin with the hair still on it—would float in the bowl. And sometimes the stuff in the bowls wouldn't be food at all; it would be corn stalks or vegetable peels or a white-flour gravy with bits of something like sawdust mixed in and flavoured with salt.

Still, the teachers would stand over the kids, with hands on their hips and threat in their eyes, and the kids knew that if they didn't force the slop down their throats, they would be beaten and maybe this would be the beating that would put them in the ground with all the other kids who had been buried around there. Their bodies would not be tricked, though: even after dinner, sometimes Maggie would faint from hunger because the mush had no nutrition and her body was still starving. In the summers, Maggie and the others would go home and get healthy again on game and fish and blueberries. And then, inevitably, relentlessly, autumn would come around again and they would be hauled back to the Mush Hole where they would force non-food down their throats and starve.

Some Mush Hole kids did see a nurse again before the end of the year. Not because they were sick—kids regularly died there from tuberculosis or measles, all without ever seeing a nurse. But some kids, like Simon and Maggie, were sent to a hospital to recover from beatings. Beatings of one kind or another were the main thing that broke up the monotony. Kids expected to have their ears boxed or to be swatted around the head, especially the back of the head where they couldn't see it coming, pretty much every week. There was a special small strapping room by the office and in it were two kinds of straps, one thin like a whip and one wide and flat that left a red mark on the skin outlining the shape of it every time it hit. The staff would take a kid into the room, close the door so there could be no escape, and strap the child on bare skin again and again. Simon was strapped because the counsellor mistook a patch of dark skin for dirt and thought he hadn't washed his hands. Maggie was strapped for speaking Cree—even in the first days of school when she didn't know any words that weren't Cree—and she was strapped for being so hungry that she picked an apple from the neighbour's tree and ate it. And sexual abuse, well, that was just part of a regular day. Everyone knew it was happening. Sometimes the principal would take a young boy or girl on his lap and molest him or her right there. There was also a counsellor, a man. At night he would stroll between the rows of kids sleeping in their beds—and suddenly a kid would begin to scream and everyone would know that counsellor was at it again, sexually abusing another kid.

There were even stories of ritual abuse and torture. Years before, one of the older Mohawk students had seen the blood marks on the floor where a kid had been beaten to death. Other students had had their arms tied to water pipes or beams above their heads, and they would be beaten like that, along their exposed torsos—but neither Maggie nor Simon ever experienced those things. They would hear the stories only after they were grown.

One of Simon's trips to the hospital happened when he was eleven years old. He stepped outside of school bounds and a counsellor, a big old man with huge hands, slapped him forcefully across the head and ears. Usually, when that sort of thing happened, the pain would go away after a day or two. But over the next few days, Simon's ear and head hurt more and more. Infection was setting in. After a week he was taken to the Six Nations Clinic: his eardrum had been broken.

Even though the wounds were shocking, and even though the doctors at the clinic could see in their examination that Simon had obviously been abused, they didn't ask any questions; they just treated the infection and transferred him to a city hospital in Brantford. The hospital wasn't any better. The nurses and doctors there offered no comfort or kindness. They looked after his bandages and made sure he had food and went to the bathroom and they kept him safe while he slept, but nothing more. They transferred him to a hospital in Amos to heal a bit more. By then it was time for summer break, so Simon went home. In the fall, he was back in the Mush Hole.

One of the worst things about living in a place like the Mush Hole is that people who are abused, who never get a rest from fear, will sometimes forget how to treat other people well. Sometimes they will even do to other people the things that have been done to them. Some of the older Mohawk youth, who had been there for a while and had survived all kinds of agonies, became bullies who terrorized younger kids. And when the new younger kids were Cree and not Mohawk, well, then the bullying was that much more intense. So the youngest Mush Hole kids who most needed comfort couldn't find it even amongst the other students.

Simon entered the Mush Hole at age 10 and stayed until he was 12 and Maggie entered at age 5 and stayed until she was about

12. There was nothing there *for* them, not even proper schooling. Each day could be endured only because one day summer would come and they could go home. Some of the kids from other nations weren't allowed even that; they had to live there year 'round. In the history of the world, surely time never moved more slowly than it did for kids in the Mush Hole.

Many years later, in 2010, stories and news articles began to surface of investigators finding tools of torture at the Brantford Mohawk Institute, and of Institute administrators ordering topsoil to cover mass graves of Indigenous children. Survivors were not surprised at what they were hearing and reading. Any time a kid had disappeared, the teachers had said "Oh, he ran away," or "Her grandma came and took her home." Of course the kids had known that the teachers were lying. Of course they had known that the school would never permit a grandmother to take a child home.

Life at home wasn't easy either. Most Cree parents had gone through residential school themselves and they had some idea of what their kids were going through. Maggie's parents could see by the vivid scars and gaunt frames that she and her brothers were being badly mistreated. They knew, too, that many children had died in the Mush Hole and that Maggie might well be the next little corpse buried on those grounds. Every August, Maggie could see the sadness on their faces. They would say "Go to school" and tell the older kids to look out for them—but Maggie could see they didn't want her to go. In the end what choice did they have? How could they possibly fight off Indian Affairs who came and scooped their small children away? After the kids had gone, the village would always be deathly quiet for a few days as the parents mourned. They had to turn to something and so they turned to alcohol. It helped.

In Simon's house in the summers, there were troubles too. First his father's feet were sore. And then they got infections that didn't heal. And then one of his legs was amputated up to the knee. After that, the atmosphere at home changed. His father, now in a wheelchair, couldn't do all the things he had once done, and his mother didn't like that. And her health problems were just getting worse and worse. The house filled with their frustration.

In fact, what was happening to both of Simon's parents was diabetes. Diabetes was consuming his father's feet, and it had brought the heart disease that eventually killed his mom. But they didn't understand diabetes. By the time they learned what they could do to make it better, it was too late; they were already very sick. Years later, Simon would be bothered by this fact: his parents had not learned in time about all the things they could do to keep their diabetes under control.

His dad coped with his changed life by doing things with his hands. He had always been a good cook. When he still had both legs, he had cooked feasts for the entire village. Now he began to cook from his wheelchair, making big meals, whipping up bannock and prepping roast goose from his wheelchair and sliding them into the oven to bake. He also took up wood carving. He had a stack of birch wood in his bedroom, which he carved with a curved blade into animals and bowls and things. His bedroom became a workshop (Simon's sister was always cleaning up sawdust) and eventually he sold his carvings in an arts and crafts store.

One year, when autumn came around, Simon was not taken to the Mush Hole but to a school in La Tuque. It was still a residential school, still a prison, still desperately lonely, but for Simon it was so much better than the Mohawk Institute that he could hardly believe it. La Tuque was a real school. The children were taught by real teachers who expected them to learn. They were sent to bed in the evenings at 10 PM, after an evening of homework and chores and exercise instead of being locked away at 7 PM as Simon had been in the Mush Hole. La Tuque had actual activities for students.

Canoeing, camping, swimming, walks, hockey, hockey, hockey. The hockey equipment was something of a joke—kids had to share hockey sticks that should have been kindling years earlier and the blades of their skates had been sharpened so many times there was hardly any blade left. Still their hockey team was so good that the local white-skinned hockey teams tried to shut the native team out of the league. It was so good that people talk about it even today.

In this environment, Simon excelled. In 1966, he had excelled in so many different sports that he won Athlete of the Year. And the next year, 1967, he did it again. Of course La Tuque was a residential school. Of course there was abuse. But there were not nearly as many cases and they were not nearly as bad as those in Brantford. Of course it was terrifying, especially for the younger kids who didn't understand what was happening. And of course there were bullies. But Simon had learned from the best Mush Hole bullies and he knew how to bully right back.

Things got better for Maggie too. She was sent to high school in Rouyn-Noranda. She still had to be separated from her brother and other people she loved, and she still had to stay in boarding homes where she was treated like a second-class citizen. And after all those years of abuse and fear, depression came to her in waves. But there was more for her in Rouyn-Noranda than threat and violence: enough food, proper teachers, real opportunities to learn. She learned well enough to be accepted to a good college in Ottawa where she studied Secretarial Sciences for one and a half years.

Maggie and Simon had done the unthinkable. They had left the Mush Hole behind.

But really, can anyone ever leave something like the Mush Hole behind? Can anyone ever really get beyond it? The physical trauma alone took decades of recovery time. Both Maggie and Simon had such extensive eardrum damage that, over the next twenty years, they each needed several surgeries to patch their eardrums back together. Their surgeons asked them to bring old medical records so that they could be certain about the treatments and medications they had received as children during their stays in the Six Nations Clinic and the Brantford Hospital. When Maggie called the Clinic, the clerk said that there were no records of her or Simon ever having stayed there; the records had been destroyed. And when she called the Brantford Hospital, the lady on the other end of the phone line said the same thing: records from more than ten years ago had been destroyed, and there were no records of Maggie or Simon or any residential school students from those years.

But Simon had been in a hospital in Amos after his stay in Brantford, and Maggie had stayed in the Val-d'Or hospital before being sent back to the Mush Hole. The Amos hospital and the Val-d'Or hospital served Cree communities; they did not need to destroy incriminating documents. They had all the information, along with the records of extensive abuse, that Maggie and Simon needed.

And then there was the emotional trauma. Maggie and Simon worked hard to put memories of the Mush Hole away and out of their lives, but, still, memories haunted them. Maggie would be at the store or going for a walk and she would see a child being frightened by something or someone, and then without warning she would be back in the office at the Mush Hole, not just remembering but reliving an assault, feeling every fist and slap and strap all over again. The depression that had started at age 12 kept coming and sometimes overwhelmed her so badly that she could hardly get out of bed. She had come this far, though, and she wanted to live her own life, not the one her abusers had wanted for her. She kept going and worked with a psychologist to heal her emotional wounds. It took a long time, years and years, and a great deal of effort. And sometimes, even now, depression sneaks up on her and takes her off guard.

Simon tried to erase the bad days of his past by drowning them in alcohol and drugs, and working in sawmills and at other temporary jobs to support his habit. Maggie and Simon met properly around this time, and Simon told Maggie she ought to be careful around him—he had a serious substance abuse problem. Maggie knew intimately the strength of Mush Hole memories and the ways they hooked a person's brain. She took him still, and looked after him as he gradually reduced his drug and alcohol dependence and sobered up. This too was a long, slow recovery.

Even three years after his last high, Simon had episodes in his sleep—he would be completely paralyzed, sweating so ferociously he would soak the sheets, his mind racing and his head throbbing in pain. Then his heart would slow again and he would fall back asleep. One night, during an episode, Simon prayed to the Creator, who had helped him get sober, to end these episodes. He felt the Creator touch him and the touch spread through his whole body. It reminded him of the angel that had met him above the clouds years before. That was his last night sweat. After that, Simon began to take his faith more seriously.

And then other health problems began to show up. In the late '80s, Simon was out on the territory, stake-claiming with a friend. Snowshoes strapped on, he was trudging through the snow, and he was thirstier than he had ever been in his life. He had no energy at all. Sure, he had gone a bit soft around the gut, but he was still an athletic man whose body had always done what he had told it to do. Now he had to guzzle jug after jug of juice just to keep going, and his friend was up ahead waiting for Simon to catch up. During his next check-up in Val-d'Or, Simon asked his doctor about it, the hospital ran some tests, and the doctor told him he had diabetes. On his way out, Simon got some pills from the nurse who suggested briefly that he might want to watch what he ate and exercise more.

One summer, about ten years ago, Maggie and Simon were out in the bush with their daughter and grandkids for a summer holiday. Their grandson's eczema flared up badly, so Maggie drove him into town to the clinic where a nurse looked after the boy—and noticed that Maggie was very pale. She tested some blood and they discovered that her hemoglobin, which should have been around 120, was at 36. Maggie was severely anemic. The clinic sent her to Amos in an ambulance for treatment and her grandson and the rest of her family followed the ambulance to Amos. She lay in the hospital for three weeks as they injected her with iron to raise her hemoglobin levels. Not long after that, the doctors discovered she needed a hysterectomy. In one of her check-ups after the surgery, Maggie learned that she too had diabetes. She wasn't too surprised— her mother had died of diabetes. And all those years of starvation and abuse in the Mush Hole had certainly affected her body's ability to process food.

Now, after Maggie and Simon both had endured cycles of starvation, they both lived with the very disease that had killed their parents. Once again, they had to obsess about food. Years earlier their parents had eaten bannock and jam by the plateful and as they ate they had wished out loud that there was something they could do to manage their diabetes; no one ever told them that the bannock and jam were making it worse. When Simon was diagnosed, the nurse had given him very little information, but he had studied on his own—in books, in libraries, in diabetic cooking classes—and, in his work as First Responder for the Ambulance Services, he was around many other people who had diabetes. By the time of Maggie's diagnosis fifteen years after his own, he knew quite a bit about the disease, much more than their parents had known, and he was fed up with feeling sick. He and Maggie talked it over. They were not helpless kids in the Mush Hole. They could take charge of their diets, of their lives. They could help themselves.

They both began to walk several kilometres a day, soon realizing that a walk out on the land was better for both mind and sugar levels than a walk around the track. And Simon, who did most of the cooking, overhauled the family kitchen. No more desserts or bannock or potatoes that made blood sugar spike and more traditional game meats and fish that made them feel better immediately. He became choosy at feasts and ate the moose or beaver meat but left the gravy in the pot. Thickened with flour, the gravy made his blood sugar spike. He blended smoothies out of spinach and blueberries and flaxseeds and cinnamon and drank them for breakfast. He ate nuts by the handful and experimented with natural blood sugar controls he had read about—like raw onions or cinnamon or lime squeezed into water or apple cider vinegar sweetened with honey. (His grandchildren thought his food experiments were a bit weird.) When Maggie revelled in the occasional comfort of a piece of bannock with raisins, Simon didn't want even a bite. The inevitable blood sugar spike wasn't worth the pleasure. Besides, what could possibly taste better than whitefish sprinkled with a few spices, cooked over an open flame, and served with greens and cucumber tossed in olive oil? Only when they were out in the bush, where every part of every day included some kind of exercise, only then did Simon enjoy a piece of bannock or dessert. Maggie worked at her diet too. She carefully taught their grandchildren about diabetes and healthy eating, and she ate what Simon cooked—but she wasn't as strict. Sometimes a piece of bannock was absolutely worth the pleasure.

Maggie and Simon were no longer young. They had come through more trauma than most people could even begin to imagine, let alone endure. But the hardest thing of all was yet to come. In 2004, the remaining Cree survivors who had attended the Brantford Mohawk Institute chartered a bus to Brantford. They would step again onto that blood-soaked soil to face what had happened to them there. It was an extraordinarily difficult thing to do.

Some people sat in the bus all the way there and, when they finally arrived, they couldn't step off the bus and go inside. Others became physically ill when the bus rolled onto the Mush Hole grounds. Maggie and Simon stepped off the bus and, with wet faces and racing hearts, they walked again through the dorms and bedrooms and dining rooms.

Everywhere, scenes came flooding back. Here, Maggie had been strapped within an inch of her life. There, Simon had been brutally assaulted. Here Maggie's ears had been boxed until they bled. There, Simon had stood paralyzed, too terrified to move. Around every corner, down every corridor were reminders that, as lonely as each of them had felt, there had been hundreds of children who had experienced exactly the same things. Written on the brick wall at the back of the school was name after name of Mush Hole students, names of people that Simon knew, names of kids who had also been afraid and mistreated. "Please help me," a child had scrawled onto the brick at the back of the school and right there, decades later, her desperation still cried out. Simon read it and his heart broke open, and years of pain deep inside awakened again.

One of the other men on the bus spoke of his hatred for the people who had abused the small boy he had once been. "I will take it to the grave," he said. Maggie and Simon understood. They had hated too. Hatred had pushed Simon into substance abuse and had left him a broken man with much personal work to do. And hatred had played a role in Maggie's relentless depression.

But Maggie and Simon didn't want to take hatred to the grave. They had come back for another reason. They were going to forgive the people who did those heinous things. Not because the abusers wanted forgiveness—that they deliberately destroyed records meant they probably had no remorse. Forgiveness wouldn't have mattered to them. Maggie and Simon had to forgive for themselves, for their own healing, so that they could finally let the Mush Hole go.

They stood in that place of fear and they prayed. First, they prayed to the Creator for their own healing of old wounds. And then they prayed for forgiveness—to forgive their tormentors, and to forgive themselves for the ways they had learned from the bullies and had hurt other people.

A few years later, Simon attended a gathering of Six Nations survivors and some of the old Mush Hole stories came up again. They hurt less this time and Simon knew the prayers had been heard and he really had healed.

Forgiveness is a tricky word; it sounds like an easy thing to do but sometimes it's the hardest, the very hardest choice to make. Sometimes it takes everything out of you to make that choice. And Simon and Maggie made it.

This is a story about two people, Maggie and Simon, from the small town of Waswanipi, Québec. When the humidity is high and the sun is up, Maggie and Simon feel it in their ears, in the places where their eardrums once broke and healed, and they know that the weather lady will say there's a low-pressure system moving over James Bay tonight, it's time to settle in for some weather.

3

The Story of Annette Spencer of Whapmagoostui

ANNETTE shot the puck and—splat. Her feet whipped out from under her and back she fell onto the ice. How unglamourous. On her back, she looked up at the ceiling lights and laughed quietly to herself. The arena was filling with sound.

Slowly she got to her feet. Her teammates were rushing at her, their arms up in victory.

"Who scored?" she asked.

"You did!" they said.

"Ummm. Are you sure?"

She couldn't believe it. A Great Moment in Hockey had just gone by, and she hadn't even seen it.

A few minutes later, Annette slumped onto the dressing room bench, still smiling from her goal, and waited for her breath to slow. Her thighs burned from the skating and every inch of her— socks, underwear, hair—was drenched in sweat. She never noticed minor discomforts during a game. She pulled off her helmet, bent to loosen her skates, and began to peel off the soggy layers of her uniform.

Those days, when she had been an athlete, they had been the best days of her life.

Annette had been thinking about those days. With a stick in her hand and skates on her feet, the puck had been easy to control. It went where she wanted it to go. And when it didn't and they lost the game—no big deal, it was all in fun anyways. A chance to hang out with the girls. She lay back on her bed, hands resting on her legs. The rigid thigh muscles had long ago softened. With each baby she had lost muscle tone and gained weight, but that wasn't the worst of it. She could hear the baby, her third, gurgling over in the other room. Annette had just finished breastfeeding and she had cried through the whole feeding. Finally, she had asked her husband to take their daughter away, into the other room, because she was afraid of what might happen to herself or to the baby. She wouldn't hurt anyone, of course, but, even though Annette could still remember every painful contraction of the birth, her body seemed not under her control, and the baby seemed like someone else's baby. She knew it was just part of her post-partum depression, or PPD, the especially intense depression that some women get after they have babies. But knowing that didn't make her feel better. All confidence was gone. That was the worst of it.

Annette knew other women with PPD. For them it had lasted a few weeks. For Annette it had been almost a year already. Her mom had helped out with the first baby, but she lived a flight away in Chisasibi and couldn't help her now. Thankfully, Annette's husband was great with babies. He was the kind of guy who helped out with the care of kids and not just with the making of them. But she could never have another baby, not like this. Nothing could be worse than living in this clamp of fear again.

She reached across to her side table and opened the drawer. She had a bag of chips in there.

Annette wanted to talk to a psychologist, but what psychologist lived way up in Whapmagoostui?

She began to think it through. Postpartum depression wasn't a new thing. Women had been getting sick—and healing—from it since long before psychologists existed. The old Cree women had used Talking Circles to manage PPD in centuries past. Annette had always bottled her feelings. She felt so isolated these days that it seemed weird even to think about talking, and there weren't any regular Talking Circles in Whapmagoostui just now.

But she didn't need a Circle to talk, she just needed to talk.

Tentatively, she tried it out on her husband, saying the words, telling him how she felt, even though he could probably see it.

Then, she talked to the friends she trusted.

The more she talked, the less alone she felt. Even her kids helped and said insightful things that could ease her from one day into the next. With time and talking, Annette managed to change her ways of thinking about things, the post-partum depression lessened, and her life fell into a natural rhythm again.

Six years passed. Annette had a fourth baby, and that sickening PPD took her over, debilitated her. With plenty of personal work and talking, she climbed out of it again.

And then a fifth baby. Sure enough, soon after the birth, there came the PPD once more, as reliable as winter following autumn. But this time, Annette wasn't the only one who was sick: the baby had been born with a tumour in her lung. Both of them were medevacked down to Montréal where the doctors operated to remove it.

As terrifying as it all was, the surgery went well and the baby was healing. But when it came time to breastfeed, Annette wasn't allowed to hold the baby to her chest. Instead, she opened her shirt, half-climbed over the railings of the infant hospital bed, and sort of dangled her breast between the tubes and wires and into the mouth of her daughter. She held perfectly still, in that awkward position, taking care not to jostle the wires, until the baby had finished feeding. There was a tube coming from a hole in the baby's chest and draining her lung, another tube coming from between her legs to carry urine away, and another tube pumping intravenous fluids into a vein in her tiny arm. As she had years earlier, Annette cried through the whole feeding, this time with worry for her sick daughter. She held out her finger for the baby to curl her hand around and know her mom was there. Post-partum depression plus being in a Montréal hospital a thousand kilometres from her husband and family plus a baby with holes cut into her and tubes snaking out—this was a whole new level of anxiety.

Annette closed up her bra and fastened her shirt. She took a tissue from the box on the hospital bedside table and wiped her eyes. She planted a kiss on her finger and touched it to her daughter's tiny forehead. Then she turned and walked down to the hospital cafeteria. She had seen on the menu board that they'd be serving orange-pineapple cheesecake today. A piece of that and she'd feel a whole lot better.

The baby recovered and Annette took her home to Whapmagoostui. Life eased again into a normal natural rhythm. The baby's scars faded.

Over the next ten years she grew into an athlete, like Annette had been, always running, always skating, always moving. If there was a sport, she wanted to play it.

Sometimes Annette would say "Slow down BB Gow! You're missing part of your lung!"

And she'd say "Sure Mom. Can you kick that ball back to me?" Annette would kick it back and smile.

"You know, Annette," her husband said one day, standing behind her and pulling her back into his chest as they watched their daughter together. "I saw a sign on the board at the sports complex. The Women's Hockey League is looking for players."

"I can't," Annette said. "I'm too busy, I don't have time."

He didn't answer. He knew that Annette worked afternoons and evenings and Saturdays. He worked just as hard. Life in Whapmagoostui, 200 kilometres beyond the last connecting road, was ridiculously expensive. Groceries especially—a small pack of frozen chicken wings was over $30, and they'd need at least three packs for a single family meal. A small head of broccoli could be over $5 and they would need three for a meal. And their trips into the bush twice a year always cost so much—they had to charter a plane to get to their land—but life on the land was an important thing for their kids to know. Even with two incomes and renting a house from the band at a good price, they could hardly manage. Annette loved sports, she missed them, but she couldn't make money playing hockey.

If her doctor were there, watching Annette's daughter play and listening to her excuses, he would probably throw up his hands in despair. "Annette," he would say, "Have fun for a few hours! Your worries will still be here." At every one of her check-ups, he worried aloud about her high risk of getting diabetes. She had had gestational diabetes, she was pre-diabetic now, and there was something in the family that was probably diabetes.

Annette couldn't be sure diabetes ran in her family because no one ever said anything about it. One of her sisters injected something that looked like it might be insulin but she had never told Annette what it was. Another sister regularly took pills for some-thing, Annette didn't know what. And their mom took some kind of pill too—Annette thought it might be a pre-diabetes pill but again she didn't know. They never talked about their medications and Annette never asked. It wasn't like pregnancy and childbirth, where they talked and giggled about every uncomfortable, smelly, messy detail. You didn't just *talk* about diabetes.

Annette didn't talk about her Sight either. When someone in the family was about to die, Annette would have a certain dream and would know a death was coming. The dream never told her who it would be, but, each time she had it, someone she loved died soon after. Her Sight had never been wrong. The Cree called it a gift, an ability to see into the world beyond this one. Annette didn't see it as a gift. The last time the warning dream came to her, she had panicked. What if her wonderful husband died? Or one of her kids? Or one of her parents? Overwhelmed with sadness before anything even happened, she had slid again into a deep depression. The person who died a few weeks later was her grandmother, 96 years old, peacefully, because it was her time. Annette's panic and sadness had been for nothing. The emotional cost of her gift was more than she had to give.

She watched their daughter wind up and send the broom-ball flying across the yard, and she felt her husband's chest behind her. Even just thinking about her Sight—Annette had to slide out from under his arms and run and get a cookie.

More time passed. Annette knew she should eat better, exercise more, take time for herself. She wanted to do each one of those things but they were so unrealistic. She was still working two jobs to make ends meet. She worried that her depression might be returning. She never had time to cook traditional foods because they took all afternoon. And, even though her husband encouraged her to get back into hockey or to go with him to the gym, it had been a long time since she had played any sports. When it came to looking after herself, life had a way of interfering. Other things were always more urgent.

One spring day in 2013, Annette came home from the clinic where she had had her annual physical. On the table in her kitchen she set a small bottle of pills and a stack of pamphlets, and then she started her computer, sat down, and began to read.

When her husband came home from work a couple of hours later, she was still there, sitting at the table, pamphlets spread around, and the internet browser open to medical websites.

"What's all this?" he asked.

"I told the doctor about having to pee in the night," she said.

"Lots of people pee in the night."

"Yeah, well, I usually don't unless I'm pregnant. And I'm not pregnant—"

"We could do something about that," he grinned at her.

"—so the doctor did some tests. I have diabetes now."

His grin faded and he sat down.

They talked late that night. About traditional foods and how long they took to cook, about whether they could stay in the bush, where the food and exercise were automatically healthier, for longer periods of time. More time in the bush meant they could get income security, but it also meant taking time away from their jobs. They drafted budgets and talked about ways of managing it. (OK, maybe the satellite TV didn't *have* to come to the bush...) They'd have to go further, though. Exercise every day. Cut back on sugar and flour and salt, read labels, count carbohydrates and calories and all that.

Annette looked down at the pamphlets strewn across the table, at the medical websites open in her browser, at her husband sitting there and writing something down. Changing the way she ate, the way she even thought about food, the times she chewed on something without thinking or reached for the comfort of junk food because eating was an easy way to manage bad feelings—these would be difficult changes to make. They would affect her whole life. And, even with everything she had read online that evening and with the doctor's warnings about how serious diabetes could be, she was actually more concerned that depression might return than about how diabetes could ravage a body. Really, thinking about depression *and* about making so many changes? She couldn't even hold it all in her head. It was overwhelming.

But—if it were only two things. She could do two things.

By the time Annette and her husband finally went to bed that night, they had decided. First, they would have more caribou and goose and ptarmigan. Over the next days, Annette gave her husband cooking lessons. She taught him how to slow-cook caribou stew and how to roast a goose and how to make ptarmigan soup. His work schedule was different than hers and he could keep an eye on the oven in the afternoons. He didn't mind at all. He even had his own favourite recipes from his childhood.

Second, hockey. She would have to be realistic. Travelling tournaments were out of the question, she was too busy. But local games, skating at the arena down the road until her gear was drenched and her legs shook from exhaustion, she would figure out a way to make time for those.

Later that week, Annette pulled her skates out of the back storage room, wiped off the dust, and set them by the door. Next time she was running errands, she would get the skates sharpened and swing by the sports complex to sign up. Great Moments in Hockey were waiting to happen.

4

The Story of Varley Mianscum
of Oujé-Bougoumou

VARLEY opened the front door of the elder's lodge in Oujé-Bougoumou, and waved a quick hello to his brother who was working there. He headed over to the lounge where his dad sat in a wheelchair with some of his friends and showed him a painting he had made. The elders all nodded at him and continued talking. They were talking about Goose Break of course. It'd be in a few weeks. The geese were just beginning to land on the lake on their way back up north. These old guys had been looking up in the sky and watching the flocks return all week. Every one of them wanted to be out in a duck blind, shooting at birds as they returned from the South.

Sure, Varley knew about the traditional ways. Hunting, fishing, chopping wood and hauling water, living in cabins and teepees in the bush. When he was a kid, his parents had lived in the bush. Varley would move in with his sister in Chibougamau during the school months, but still he spent quite a bit of time on the land. Even now, grown, working and living in Oujé-Bougoumou, he and his boyfriend would sometimes go hunting on the weekends. Shoot a partridge and roast it up for dinner. (Well, his boyfriend would come along, but he wouldn't hunt.) Or they would take his boy-friend's daughter and her friends to the bush camp for the weekend. It was fun. Varley was up for bush camp as much as the next guy. His mom had said to him once, a few years back, "Traditional food is good for people with diabetes, Varley. You should probably eat more of it." That was how Varley had found out that she knew he had diabetes. She was smart, she had probably known for a while. And sure, he loved a plate of moose or goose now and then.

But. Hiding quietly, without moving, in a blind for hours to shoot down geese from above? Or beetling an ATV through black flies and muskeg and underbrush to follow a big honking moose, shooting the thing without missing, gutting and bleeding and field dressing it, and then hauling it back home, out of the truck and up the front stairs and into the kitchen to butcher it there on the table, smelling up the house until he got all the pieces into the freezer? Oh man, that just wasn't his life. Life on the land was what guys like his dad wanted. It sounded like way too much effort.

What Varley wanted was variety. Oudjé-Bougoumou had really only one kind of food. Maybe two—traditional food and what you could get at the corner store or diner. But for six years Varley had lived in Montréal, working for Cree Patient Services on rue Ste-Catherine. Most things about Montréal (crowds, traffic, summer heat) he didn't miss. But restaurants. What he would do for more restaurants in Oujé. Real restaurants, mind you, not Tim Horton's. One with Chinese food, one with Thai food, one Mexican, one Italian, and one high-end fine dining restaurant. Oh, and maybe a couple of stores for shopping: an electronics store, a proper movie store with plenty of selection, and a clothing store or two. That'd be about right. Actually, that'd be perfect.

The other thing Varley wanted was to take it easy. He had always been good at avoiding conflict. When he was a boy in school in Chibougamau, he was exactly the kind of kid who would have been bullied. He was Cree, he didn't want to speak French, he was taller than his peers, and somehow he was different but he didn't yet know he was gay—other kids were bullied for much less. But, even then, Varley could smell confrontation coming. If he saw kids arguing on the school yard, or ganging up on one person for some stupid reason that never made sense, or if he saw someone he thought might want to take a swing at him, Varley would go someplace else. Hang out with his friends for a while, or go home to watch TV, or just walk quietly to a different corner of the schoolyard. He would go to wherever conflict wasn't. Some people said he was an old soul.

His dad settled back in his chair and started chatting about his youth again, about what life was like when he grew up. After a while, the orderly came over with a tray and a syringe and insulin. The old man lifted his shirt, the orderly passed the needle to him, and he injected himself into his stomach. The orderly left. Then someone farted and the old guys went off on a round of jokes about that. His dad was such a joker. There was nothing he liked better than to make people laugh. Varley laughed along.

He loved these guys. Their lives had been something else— some had lived on the land, some had gone through residential school, some had raised kids or worked all kinds of jobs. More recently, they coped with all the ways in which bodies get old. And diabetes had affected a few of them. Years back, diabetes had been tremendously stressful, almost a death sentence. His dad had been diagnosed about ten or fifteen years ago. He'd been healthy for a while and then he had started getting sick with one thing or another until his kidneys gave out. Eventually he had moved into the elder's lodge because Varley and his mom couldn't do the required daily care by themselves.

There had been a time in Varley's early thirties, a few years after his own diabetes diagnosis, when he had controlled the disease with diet and exercise. He walked regularly then and headed to the gym on days he didn't walk. He ate carefully—more traditional meats, fewer packaged soups and pastas and TV dinners, fewer doughnuts and less junk food—and it paid off. His blood sugar levelled off, he had more energy, he didn't need any meds, his blood pressure went down, even his mood improved. He felt better, no question.

But it took so much effort. So much vigilance. Varley had to stab himself with a lancet and test his blood sugar in the glucometer five or six times a day just to stay on top of it. He had to think about every tiny bite that went into his mouth; he could never just eat. And exercising every day, even more if the glucometer numbers were too high—it had sounded like an easy thing to do. But actually scheduling the time to move his body, and then getting up off the couch when it was really the only place he wanted to be, or giving up part of an evening of hanging out with his friends or watching Netflix or HBO to go for a walk—it felt like the glucometer ran his life. It made his life *about* diabetes. He didn't want to set goals to bring down his sugar levels and then stress out over not reaching them. He didn't want to have to think about disease all the time. His life was about so much more than that.

And so Varley let go. He let go of the vigilance and the policing and the rigid schedule. He let go of the effort of maintaining fitness and a traditional diet. It meant that he had to be extra careful with his pills if he didn't want to feel sick. It meant that he had to go onto insulin—which was, admittedly, inconvenient; he always had to haul the stuff around and calculate how much to inject. And it meant that, after a while, his blood sugar levels started to seesaw. When they were really low, he would get lightheaded and the room would start to spin. When they were really high, like above 20, he would be so tired he couldn't do any work. But being careful with pills and insulin took much less out of him and was less stressful than monitoring everything he ate and staying fit and having to think constantly about diabetes.

His dad had always said, "If you have a headache, just don't think about it. It'll probably go away." Diabetes couldn't be like a headache; once you had it, it was always there. But it didn't have to run his life. He saw people at the clinic with diabetes who were really young and that was concerning, especially when so many of the kids were Cree. But it wasn't the death sentence it had once been. If Varley felt like it, he could pack up his pills and insulin and fly to Thailand if he wanted to.

It was time for his dad's dinner. Varley wheeled him around to the dining room table, gave him a hug and a kiss on the cheek and said goodbye, and walked home. He checked his phone. His boyfriend had texted. They were invited over to a friend's place later that evening to watch a movie. And his mom had left a message— could Varley please swing by the corner store and pick up some vegetable oil? It was pork chops and onions for dinner.

Stories We Heard Along the Way: Fire

Once, a house in Mistissini caught fire. The fire department in Chibougamau sent a firetruck, but it missed the turnoff at Mistissini and drove on to Lake Albanel. The fire department sent a second fire truck then, and it didn't miss the turnoff—but it turned so quickly that it ended up in the ditch. The third vehicle to leave Chibougamau was the fire chief's truck. It reached the site of the fire first. By the time the firetrucks finally got there, the house had burned down.

·

At La Tuque Residential School, one very young boy was repeatedly punished for bedwetting. And to make matters worse, each time he wet his bed he would have to carry the wet sheets to the laundry the next morning, in front of the whole school. It was so humiliating. The other boys in his dorm didn't like this and decided to do something. One day, in the early morning, when their bladders were full, every 6- to 8-year-old boy in the dorm, 26 boys in all, got out of bed, dropped his pants, and peed onto his own mattress. Then all 26 of them carried their wet bedding to the laundry in front of the whole school, and the boy who was always punished wasn't alone. In 2006, the La Tuque school was razed to the ground in a great big fire. Nobody cried.

·

Much to the chagrin of Public Health and Safety, the firehall in one of the communities caught fire one day. The firemen didn't want to lose the expensive fire truck along with the building, and so someone ran inside to drive the fire truck out of the burning building—only to find that the truck was out of gas. In the end, a group of people came running and helped to push it.

•

The Eastmain summer forest fire of 2013 was so intense that the power went down everywhere in northern Quebec. The access road to the town of Eastmain had flames on both sides.

•

One of the communities was looking to have someone teach wood-stove safety. It turned out that a relative of the fire chief had the proper training and got the job. Shortly after he came up north and moved into the community, his own house partly burned down—from a woodstove fire.

5

The Story of Sandra Judith Bulluck*
of Whapmagoostui

SANDRA Judith Bulluck's grandfather attended church on Sunday mornings. He listened to the sermon and sang the songs and prayed the prayers. Then he came home and sat on his bed. Sandra sat beside him.

"I don't believe everything that minister said," he would say to her. "I know from my own life and the lives of my people on the land—some of those things are not true."

The next Sunday, he went back to church.

Years later, Sandra heard a story from an elder:

In the earliest times of colonization, a missionary said to a Cree elder, "That drum you have—it has the devil in it!"

"The devil?" the elder asked. "Here in my little drum?"

"Yes!" the missionary said. "Burn the drum."

So the elder threw his drum on the bonfire and watched it burn to ash.

Then he turned to the missionary. "It's okay now," he said. "I have killed your devil for you. You don't have to worry about him anymore."

*Names and details in this story have been changed to protect identities.

And then the elder went home and made himself another drum.

Things happen that you can't control. Sometimes you gotta do what you gotta do, but always you can have your own mind. You don't have to take things lying down. This is what Sandra learned from her grandfather and from the elder.

It was karaoke night in town. Sandra's friend stomped and swayed and sang on stage, the audience clapped, and Sandra quietly sang along. *La la la la something arising.* She hadn't heard the song in a while and couldn't remember the words. *Ba da da something la the way.* She checked the karaoke screen—

She couldn't *see* the karaoke screen. It was right there and the words were on it, but for all the squinting and staring in the world, they were too blurry for Sandra to read. Something was wrong with her eyes.

Sandra looked back at her friend. She'd worry about her vision in the morning. It was probably something to do with menopause.

In the clinic the next morning, the medical staff ran tests. They peered into Sandra's eyes. They asked all kinds of questions. They made her pee into a cup. They did a fasting test and Sandra couldn't eat anything for twelve long hours, and then, when she was hungry, they took a vial of her blood and tested her blood sugar.

"Your guess isn't far off," the doctor said, after all the tests were done. "Your vision is blurry because you have diabetes. Menopause can trigger diabetes in some people."

Diabetes? Sandra was shocked—for about ten seconds. She had read that people who had experienced trauma or high levels of stress were more likely to get diabetes, as if the experiences and memories sucked the sweetness out of life and left blood sugar levels forever imbalanced. And she knew a thing or two about bad memories and trauma.

She looked around the little examination room. A blood pressure pump, some anatomy diagrams, tongue depressors, a tray of sterilized instruments—all the things you usually see in clinic rooms. Diabetes was serious. She might soon be in this room more than she wanted to be.

Sandra drove home from the clinic. So she was supposed to exercise more, no big deal. She liked to walk anyways. It got her out of doors and cleared her head.

And she would eat a traditional diet. Twenty years ago, that would have been a problem. Twenty years ago Sandra couldn't even clean a goose. She could clean a fish—she had watched her mom clean fish when she was younger—and she might have managed a beaver, but they hadn't taught goose-cleaning in residential school. Someone had brought her a limp-necked freshly killed goose back then, and Sandra had had to call her sister. With the phone at her ear, her sister coaching her through, Sandra had plucked the bird until it was naked and her kitchen a mess, had cut it from stomach down to butt, and had shoved her hand in there to pull out the guts—carefully because the meat would taste funny if she burst the wrong gland. She hadn't put down the phone until the goose intestines lay curled in one bowl to be eaten later, gizzard and heart and liver were in a different bowl, and a hollow bare-skinned goose roasted slowly in her oven. But that was a long time ago and these days Sandra knew her way around hunted animals and traditional foods. She would ask her sons-in-law to kill a few extra birds this year for her freezer and to catch her some fish. She'd get used to a traditional diet. She'd miss starchy foods at first, of course, but with time she'd get used to it.

But the clinic nurse said she was supposed to reduce stress. How? How do you make stress just *go away*? Some of her worst stress came from things she remembered. It didn't work to just try not to think about the things that had happened to her—memories persisted like bad heartburn. They came back to her mind and bumped into her head whether she wanted them to or not. Could you even make memories *go away*?

Once a month a therapist came through town and you could get in line to talk to her for an hour or so. An hour or two for a lifetime of memories? And to a person who might be well trained and compassionate and all that but who could never really understand what it was like to grow up Eenou in the twentieth century? That kind of therapy helped plenty of people. Sandra could see its effects in people she knew. But it didn't feel right for her.

And then she heard that her community was starting up a Talking Circle and it would be run by local elders. They were doing it the traditional way: people were going to sit in a circle, listen to one another and tell their stories, and, through the telling and the listening, recover from emotional trauma together.

That was more like it. She would start with the Talking Circle. Tell a story or two. See what it was all about.

At the Talking Circle, she talked about that time at her first residential school, an Anglican one…

Sandra threw out her chest, pumped her bare legs, and ran through the school, away from Angry Supervisor, the Supervisor with a whole row of whipping belts hanging in her closet. Down the corridor and into the kitchen where she slid under the overhang of a counter and crouched, immobile. Plonk plonk plonk—Supervisor's footsteps catching up. Sandra jumped out from her hiding spot and ran again, this time down the stairs into the playroom, and slipped silently into a locker and closed the door. Plonk plonk plonk. She ran out again, but where could she go now? The dining room! She ran there and was about to squeeze under a chair when Supervisor's huge hand closed around her arm and by the time Sandra could turn her head, the whipping belt was chewing up her back and legs again and again and again. Sandra couldn't see which whipping belt the Supervisor had chosen this time, especially for Sandra, but she could see that Angry Supervisor's lips were parted and her face looked unmistakeably satisfied.

But Angry Supervisor and Sandra were not alone. Also in that room, watching quietly without moving so that he wouldn't be noticed, was a Cree worker, a man from another community, who saw it all. Sandra spent a few days recovering, but two weeks later Angry Supervisor was gone. The girls in the dorm who knew the gossip said she had been dismissed. The Cree worker had reported her.

That was the best part of residential school. You felt close to the other Cree kids and workers. They were your kin, your family, when your real family was so far away.

And she talked about that time at another school, farther south...

Thunk. The car hit the ditch, half-turned over, and Sandra looked at the world upside down.

Oh crap.

She was fine, they were all fine. But now they wouldn't get to her friend's reserve. There was nothing to do in town. And it was so awkward there, where they were supposed to behave as if they were white. Everything about that felt wrong. Why should she pretend to be white? Why would she even want to?

The cop loaded Sandra, her friend Eva, and Eva's brother into his car. Eva's brother went back to the rez and Sandra and Eva went back to their rooming house in town. Their landlords, a European couple who thought they were doing the world a service by billeting some Cree girls, started to scold. Shame this and shame that and God didn't want you going to that reserve and see how he stopped you and blah blah blah.

Still, Sandra had planned an entire evening on the rez, whether or not she was supposed to, and had spent a whole day anticipating it. Even that much was satisfying. No matter how bad things got, they were always better if you had your own mind.

And about that other time, also at school in the South...

It was evening at Sandra's boarding house. There was a knock and Sandra's landlord answered the door. The Guidance Counsellor from Indian Affairs stepped inside. She had news for Sandra: her parents had both died in an airplane accident on the way to their trapline. The Counsellor was gentle and kind and tried to be comforting. It was a terrible thing for children to lose their parents, she said. Unfortunately Sandra would not be permitted to fly home before the end of term, not even for the funeral—Indian Affairs policy. The next day Sandra was sent to class like nothing had happened.

The sadness was overwhelming. It hurt Sandra to the bone and it lasted for months. Years. It would have been so much easier if she could have been at the funeral. Or if she could have seen her brothers and sisters who went to residential schools in other towns. Or if Sandra's sister, the only one permitted to live in the same town, could have roomed with her here at the boarding house. Then the two of them might grieve their parents and heal together—but residential school policy was to separate families as much as possible. Break the bonds.

Or try to.

And about that time, back at home in Whapmagoostui, after she was married.

Sandra had put on weight. With every baby she birthed, there was a bit more flesh around her middle. She didn't mind. What bothered Sandra was her husband's behaviour. He had met a few too many Angry Supervisors himself, he had learned from them, and he had developed a taste for beating her.

But Sandra was no skinny young thing anymore. She had some heft to her now. The next time he tried to beat her—she fought back. Hard.

He had wounds to nurse that night. And he never beat her again.

You don't have to take things lying down.

Over the weeks, then months, the stories from all the people in the Talking Circle accumulated and filled the air. Sandra and the others there saw how their own stories looked alongside the stories of everyone else. They tried to understand the people who had mistreated them and their own reactions to the abuse. With every part of the process came relief. Relief to be heard, to share with her kin, to hear stories from other people who had gone through similar things. Relief to have compassion for those people—she knew quite a few—who couldn't yet talk about all they had endured, who couldn't yet heal. And a relief to hear again what she already knew, that she had no control over other people, that memories never went away but she wasn't helpless. Always, she could have her own mind.

And with that, her diabetes became more manageable. In fact, the Talking Circles combined with Sandra's walking exercise and mostly traditional diet were so successful that, for three years, Sandra needed no diabetes medication at all.

Sandra got on with her life.

She had already finished a university degree and had been a teacher for 11 years. She had raised her six kids as best she could—not easy for anyone, even harder for residential school students who had never seen anyone be a parent—and they turned out just fine. She had spoken to elders to learn how the traditional Cree taught biology and science and chemistry and language as part of life, on the land, and not in classrooms nor through textbooks. She had separated from her husband. She had her diabetes under control.

She took a job then that had her travelling to the nine communities of Eeyou Istchee. The work was important. She was up in a plane every week, looking down on the lakes and rivers. She spent her nights in lodges and transits, meeting new people and seeing the world. It was wonderful.

It was a lot of upheaval.

It made Sandra's diabetes worse.

Travel and diabetes were not good companions. Sandra was in a different place every week with a different schedule every day—regular exercise became difficult to manage. And getting traditional food on the road was often impossible. Sometimes she would be so tired, so hungry from all the travel that she reached for pastry or juice, foods that made her blood sugar levels spike. She still went to the Talking Circles when she was home and they still helped, but life on the road was interfering with her other routines.

There's no easy cure for diabetes. You have to manage it, best you can, every meal, every day. And sometimes things happen that you can't control. Sometimes you have to do what you have to do. After a few years in her new job, Sandra had to start taking pills. After some more years, she had to take insulin too, every day.

Sandra worked at her travelling job for many years until it came time to retire.

As soon as she could, she went back to her reliable traditional diet and felt better right away; the old Cree had really understood well-being, *miyupimaatisiiun.* She started walking again too. Her health magazines had new research that probiotics help keep bodies balanced so she started taking some of those. Now that she was in town more, not on the road, she could attend sweats and other traditional ceremonies.

And of course, the Talking Circles. They had been her most important diabetes-management tool. In them, she had made sense of a complicated life and had come out the other side, happy. Little by little, her blood sugar levelled off.

The other day, she told the story of the devil in the drum again. It's up to her now to keep the stories going, to remind people that stuff happens—but you can have your own mind. You don't have to take things lying down.

What a great life.

6

The Story of Mary Niquanicappo
of Whapmagoostui

IN SPRING of 2002, Mary did all the things she usually did in spring. She cleaned the storage room, she pulled her rubber boots from the back of the closet, she laid the mud mat down by the door, and she went to the clinic for her yearly check-up. The doctor ran routine tests and sent her home. A few days later, Mary was called back to the clinic. The nurse said that her blood sugar levels were too high and gave her pills and some pamphlets. Mary, she said, had diabetes and needed to see the nutritionist next. Mary nodded and thanked the nurse. Then she listened as the nutritionist explained a few things and left, calm and composed. She walked home, as if nothing had happened, and went about her life.

Two or three days went by. Mary was cleaning up her kitchen— and the nurse's words sank in like a cleaver. *I have diabetes. People with diabetes get infections that don't heal. Their limbs are amputated and they go blind and die young. I'm 25 years old and my life is over,* she thought. She crumpled into a chair, her heart began to race, and her breathing went shallow. *Who will look after my mother and grandmother when I die?*

After a while, still terrified, Mary got up and finished cleaning the kitchen. There were things that had to be done.

Then the nightmares set in. She dreamt that she got a tiny scrape, from a kitchen knife or the raw edge on the door at the bar where she worked, and it became infected. Her skin broke and oozed pus, her limbs were sawed off, and she died a painful, messy death. In the mornings, she woke, took care of her family, went to work, and waited for the infection that would bring about the inevitable amputation, the inevitable early death. At night she came home again to more nightmares about how it would happen. For three or four years, Mary lived like this, swimming in fear and grieving what she knew to be true—that soon, any day now, she would die.

Eventually, she found work as a cleaner at the clinic. There, hanging around every day with people who knew about diabetes and seeing other people who also had diabetes, Mary learned a bit more. Managing the disease was a day-to-day thing. If she checked her skin every night and took care of any cuts, she could prevent infection. If she ate less sugar and starch and more traditional food, she could probably bring down her sugar levels. If she exercised every day, she might bring them down further. She even heard about some people who were able to manage their diabetes without pills or insulin. It didn't *have* to be a death sentence. The knot of fear in her chest gradually loosened and her nightmares stopped.

Every now and again, Mary hears about people who are devastated by their diagnosis. She really understands that.

Mary was raised mostly by her grandmother, but also by her mother. When she was in high school, sixteen years old, her mother told her to quit school and go to work. The family needed money. Mary had her own idea: she found work but she stayed in school too. Her mom was okay with that decision. As long as Mary brought money home. A few years later, though, after high school finished,

Mary wanted more than Whapmagoostui had. She wanted to leave, she wanted to study, she wanted to travel. So she bought a ticket south and she quit her job. Her mother wasn't so happy about that.

Mary's first stop was John Abbott College in Montréal, where she had decided to study Social Sciences. The city was overwhelming. It was big. It smelled awful. It was so hard to get around. Nothing worked like it had in Whapmagoostui, the rules were different. Once, she was on the metro with some idea of where she wanted to go, but she wasn't sure which train station she needed to stop at. A friendly looking man sat down beside her and she asked him for directions. He said he knew just where she was going and he would help her. In fact, he was going that way himself so he would take her there, show her the way. A few minutes later, they stepped off the train together—but Mary saw right away that something was wrong. This was not the stop she needed. He was taking her to a different area of town altogether. She tried to get away from him then, but his hand closed around her arm and he said she was coming home with him now, he had something else on his mind. She began to push back at him and call out for help. The subway platform was full of men and women and kids milling about, but no one stopped to help the little Inuit-Cree woman calling out. The kids stared silently, and the adults all looked away. Finally Mary got away from him and found her own way to the place she was looking for. After that, she never asked another passenger for help. When she needed help on the metro, she asked only the transit workers. Being careful around strangers was one of those city rules she knew now and hadn't known before.

Little by little, Mary grew to understand the city, its systems and its rhythms. She even began to love it. At the end of her school year, she decided to stay in Montréal—things at home with her mother were always a little difficult and she wasn't yet ready to go back to that. There was more to see. Mary found part-time work and was soon able to make enough money to stay in Montréal.

One day she answered an advertisement for a job that looked interesting. The job, she soon found out, wasn't really a job but an arranged marriage. A man from Pakistan wanted to be a Canadian citizen and the only way he could do that was to marry someone already Canadian. She married him and moved into his house—she slept in her own room—as he went through the citizenship process. He was a kind man who treated her well, who was good company, and who cared about her wellbeing. But after that whole process, which had taken more than a year, he still didn't qualify for citizenship or residency. He decided then to move to United States and try for residency there and he asked Mary to come with him.

She thought about it. Certainly he was a good husband and she enjoyed her life with him. But she felt too young to move to another country. She was already so far away from her northern home. And she had found work in Montréal at the Native Women's Association and she loved it. From her husband's house she packed up what she was able to carry, left her other things behind, and walked away from his home, never to see him again. (Later, she learned that he had annulled the marriage.)

Getting back to her own ways and her independence felt wonderful, and for a long time, Mary told no one at home that she had been married for 14 months. But talking about experiences helped her to understand them. Back when she had been just ten years old, and again when she was nineteen, she had been raped and talking about those experiences had siphoned off the fear and carried her through. Talking would help now too. And, if she talked about her marriage, then other women who might go through the same thing could know they weren't alone.

Mary posted on Facebook that she had been married for 14 months to a kind man from Pakistan and they had now separated because he was moving farther away. In Whapmagoostui, it was hot news, and in less than a day, everyone knew.

Mary continued working at the Native Women's Association of Montréal and eventually transitioned to working at a women's shelter there. She loved it. She loved living in Montréal. She loved working with other Indigenous women—she could understand them and they understood her. She had the freedom to do what she wanted to do. So many interesting things happened in the city, once you knew where to find them. And it was much easier to exercise. Much easier to be healthy.

After a while, she tried another year of school, this time at Dawson. In one of her courses, she was told to go to the library and research something for an essay. She took her pad of paper and went to the library. The other students were already there. They were moving around the book stacks pulling out books, getting information they needed and putting books back on the shelf. It was obvious they already knew how to research—they had been taught in high school—but her Whapmagoostui school hadn't taught her anything about research. She had never been in a library like this before. She didn't know where to begin and she was afraid to ask the librarians. Soon Mary wasn't passing her courses, and then she lost funding for school and went back to work at the shelter. Once or twice a year she would visit Whapmagoostui.

At one point, she travelled to Manitoba and stayed with an uncle there for three months. When it came time to leave, she had no money for the trip back to Québec. She thought about hitchhiking but there was that time back on the Montréal metro with the man who had tried to force her home with him… You had to be cautious around strangers.

One night Mary dreamt that she hitchhiked and reached Montréal safely. She knew then that she'd be okay, dreams could be trusted, and the next day she left to hitchhike home. Eventually, she got all the way back to Montréal, she worked for a while to earn her flight fare, and she flew to Whapmagoostui.

She had come home and she stayed.

In the first years after Mary was diagnosed with diabetes, money was tight. She worked at a few different things, taking extra hours when she could, but Whapmagoostui is an expensive town. Her mom was in the Chisasibi hospital—Mary flew there from time to time for a visit—and Mary lived with and cared for her grandmother: the costs added up. She could pay the rent and buy essentials of healthy food, soap, and things they needed around the house, but there was no money for extras like cookies or pop or potato chips.

Mary took her pills diligently. They weren't great—they made her feel uncomfortable—but her body needed them and now people needed her, so she learned to live with the discomfort. After a few years, in 2004, she got pregnant and with pregnancy her blood sugar levels were more erratic than ever. The nurse recommended that she switch to the insulin medication and taught Mary to inject herself. She felt better right away and stayed on the insulin, even after her son was born.

A few years later, she was pregnant again. (Thankfully, Whapmagoostui had Inuit men to date—Mary didn't want to date Whapmagoostui Cree men because she seemed to be related to most of them and didn't want to date a relative accidentally.) This time, with insulin, her blood sugar levels stayed even throughout the pregnancy and Mary gave birth to a baby girl. Her uncle in Manitoba had once told her about a dream that came to him one night in which Mary had birthed a girl and he had raised her as his own. So Mary gave him her new daughter to raise. Dreams could be trusted; it would be all right.

Little by little, Mary came to understand diabetes, its systems, and its rhythms. It became part of her life—like taking care of her son or her grandma. Like brushing her hair. After ten years, she couldn't even remember a time when she wasn't taking medication for her diabetes.

MARY NIQUANICAPPO

Nowadays, Mary is still taking care of people. Her mother has passed away, but she looks after her grandmother and her son, who has mild autism. They are both comfortable and rewarding relationships, they are the most important people in her life, and they both need a great deal of care. Mary puts everything she can into giving good care and can now afford to buy sweets and treats for the people she loves.

When she has her check-up at the clinic, Mary expects a big lecture from the nurses and they never disappoint. "You have to cut back on sugar," they say. They're right. It's a nice thought, cutting back on sugar. But sometimes, after a long day's work, Mary comes home and there's more to do—a mess to clean up, or a crisis to avert. Eating a cookie gives her the energy to get through those next twenty minutes of whatever needs to be done. Her diabetic body suffers as a result, yes, but sometimes, getting through those twenty minutes is more important. Sometimes there just isn't enough energy at the end of the day for anything else. (If the nurses knew, they'd probably tell her to cut back on sugar and portion sizes for her son too, but other kids get so many things her son can't have because of his autism—how can she not give him those few treats he's able to have now that she can afford them?)

"You should lose weight," they say, "exercise more." Well, yes. But in Whapmagoostui, large women are accepted and putting on weight is normal, even encouraged. It's part of the culture, Mary feels. And if someone offers you food, it's disrespectful to refuse it. As for exercise, the tradition used to be that exercise was necessary when you were out on the land, but the winter months in town were a season of rest. That norm is changing—these days you'll see locals of all shapes and ages trundling to the gym in town for Boot Camp or BounceFit, or to the arena for hockey—but it's not part of Mary's life yet.

"You should eat more traditional food, less processed food," they say. Mary agrees. She loves traditional food. She'd eat it every day if she could. But how? She doesn't have time to go hunting herself, and, if she did, she would have to bring her grandmother and son along into the bush, and both of them have fragile health and can't be far from the clinic. Sometimes she gets traditional food through Facebook—last fall someone gave her five geese—and then it's a treat for all three of them. At the community feasts, she can get traditional food too. She tries to attend every one. Unfortunately, she always has to leave early to inject insulin right after eating. It would be easiest to inject it at the feast and to stay until the end, but some people are bothered by the sight of needles and Mary doesn't want to upset them. She could inject in the bathroom, but bathrooms aren't always clean and she can't be sure a bathroom is sanitary enough for injecting. And so she enjoys her traditional food, and then rushes home to take her insulin, the wonderful taste of goose or beaver still in her mouth.

"You have to watch for emotional eating," the nurses say. Mary could write the book on emotional eating. So many things have happened in her life; she would like nothing more than to see a psychologist every week to sort out the emotional traumas that drive her to eat. But Whapmagoostui has neither a psychologist nor housing for a psychologist. Someone flies up every once in a while, and it helps for Mary to talk about things then, but she would like to talk to someone regularly and that isn't possible. So she eats.

The nurses—who are also her friends—go on about self-care. "This is serious, Mary! You have to take better care of yourself!" She's heard it so often she could *give* the lecture. She understands what the nurses are saying and she thinks they're right. If it were her son or her grandmother, she would want them to focus on self-care first, and to take care of others second. But, Mary thinks, they don't have her responsibilities. Support workers for her grandmother and son are supposed to help her out, and some of them are wonderful. But some are less dependable and, in the end, it all falls back on Mary.

Last year, she was so exhausted that she begged and pleaded with the doctors and Social Services for a short break. She arranged for her grandmother to stay with her aunt, and Mary and her son flew to Montréal, he to summer camp and she to the women's shelter for a few weeks to recover. Immediately, with some time to focus on herself, she was able to exercise more, to eat better, to sleep more deeply, and to live a healthier life. But soon the respite came to an end and they returned to Whapmagoostui. Mary was happy to be with her grandmother again, but nothing had really changed.

Mary would love to try to control her diabetes with exercise and food so that she wouldn't need medication. But that will have to wait until she has more time for herself. These days, doing all those things isn't an option. She's no longer terrified of losing a limb or dying young from diabetes. The disease doesn't control her life. And every day she works at the clinic, she's reminded again of how many others have diabetes too. She does what she can—she takes her insulin faithfully, she eats traditional food as often as she can get it, and she talks frankly about the difficult things in her life so that stress doesn't bottle up inside. It's not everything she ought to be doing, the nurses say. But for now it will have to be enough.

7

The Story of Victor Gilpin of Eastmain

ONCE upon a time, in the days before the James Bay Hydroelectric Project was built, the Eastmain River was wide and deep. It carried freshwater past the town of Eastmain and emptied into James Bay. Freshwater fish, like pike and walleye and sturgeon, swam in the river and the people of Eastmain lowered nets into the water to catch them. The water was so calm and clear that one day, when young Victor Gilpin was out checking fishnets with his mother, he saw clouds reflected in the water. All of their drinking and cooking and cleaning water came from the river too. Sometimes, when Victor's grandmother needed water in the home, she sent him to the river. If it was summertime, he carried the water in two pails attached to the ends of a pole that sat across his shoulders. If it was winter, then the people hitched their sleds to the dogs, took some buckets, and went down to the frozen river on the sled, and Victor would help them out. There would be a hole already cut into the ice where he could scoop water up into his bucket. If the hole had frozen over, Victor chipped away the thin layer of ice before dipping in his scoop and filling his pails. With the river right there, Victor and his friends always had something to do. In summer, they swam in it almost every day and would sometimes dive into the water off the end of the long dock. There was one day Victor went swimming four or five times in the same day. In winter, when the river froze, he and his friends would slide down the riverbank on their sleds, and, one winter, the older boys cleared the snow off the ice and played hockey. For Victor and the people of Eastmain, the river was their lifeblood.

But the big dam was coming. In the early 1970s, the Province of Québec began to prepare for the massive changes in the waterways and landscape that the dam for the Hydroelectric Project would bring about. The people in the town of Fort George, for instance, were relocated to Chisasibi because their island was going to be eroded by the diverted river. And the people of Eastmain were told that the Project would divert 90% of the flow and their river would not be as wide as it once was.

The day the dam began to work, however, the people of Eastmain woke up to something very different from what they expected. Overnight, the Eastmain River had lost nine-tenths of the flow, yes, but with much less water flowing downstream, the river could no longer resist the salty tides that pushed upstream from James Bay. Overnight, the great clear freshwater river that flowed by the town had slowed and narrowed and become saltwater.

The people of Eastmain struggled. Now their water was filthy, salty, undrinkable. Now the freshwater fish floated, dead, in the saltwater and could not be eaten. Now their children didn't want to swim in the stream every day as they once had and began to look around for things to do. Now the people had to collect rainwater or melt snow for their cooking and cleaning. When they ran out of water, they had to canoe out to the islands in the bay. On the islands were huge rocks with wide indentations in them that held rainwater like big stone bowls, and the people would have to collect their water there.

Today the Eastmain River is still slow and shallow and salty—but an astonishing thing has happened. The freshwater fish like pike and walleye and sturgeon have, over time, adapted to live in saltwater. In recent years, Cree fishermen have been catching those same freshwater fish that they caught years ago, but now they catch them in the saltwater river.

When Victor was six years old, he was taken away from his home beside the Eastmain River and sent to the French residential school in Fort George. Victor was a bright kid and liked to learn new stuff. Some of what he was supposed to learn in residential school, though—well, it seemed kind of pointless. It was a Catholic school, so every Sunday he and the other kids had to file into the chapel where they sat in rows on benches and were given a rosary, which was a bunch of beads on a string. The beads seemed important: the kids were supposed to touch a big bead and say one thing, and then touch the next bead on the string, a smaller bead, and say something else, and so on. If, during the chapel service, Victor whispered something to his friend sitting on the bench beside him, or even turned his head in the direction of his friend, then later a wooden meal board would be slapped down on his hands.

Something else that seemed awfully important in residential school had to do with bedsheets. In the dorm, the rooms were heated by radiators that carried boiling water from a boiler. The hot water for bathing was heated in that same boiler. One night, a young frightened boy in Victor's dorm wet his sheets as he slept. The next day, all the boys in that dorm saw the counsellor enter the bathroom and fill a bathtub. They could tell by how long the water ran that the tub had about four or five inches of water in it, and they could tell from the massive steam clouds billowing out of the bathroom that it was only hot water coming straight from the boiler. Then the counsellor sauntered out of the bathroom and, as if it were nothing at all, he picked up the boy who had wet his bed and carried him into the bathroom, closing the partition behind them. The young boy screamed and screamed and screamed. They took him away then for medical attention and, after he came back, the kids saw his skin had been badly burned to the top of his ankles. He had been made to stand in the scalding water as punishment for wetting the bed while he slept.

Another punishment for wet bedsheets involved vertical posts. Four posts held up beams that supported the roof. They were made of steel, about three or four inches in diameter, extremely strong and extremely slippery. Sometimes, boys who wet their beds were made—by the same counsellor—to climb a slippery post, up about four feet, and a mop handle was carefully positioned upright under their pajama-covered butts. The boys were supposed to stay there, gripping the slippery post, immobile for a long while. If a boy lost his grip on the post, perhaps because he was shaking with effort, or because he was tired or simply not strong enough to hold up his weight on a slippery pole for that long, that carefully positioned mop handle could really hurt him. All the while, the counsellor stood there watching, as if he enjoyed the show. To Victor and the other kids who were also watching, every minute a kid was up on the pole seemed like forever.

There were punishments for speaking Cree, for speaking at the wrong time, for eating certain foods, for not eating other foods, and on and on. There were punishments for so many things that it was hard to keep track of them. Much of the time, Victor would have given anything to be back safe at home by the Eastmain River where beads and bedsheets were not so terribly important, and where life made so much more sense.

One February, when Victor was nine years old and had been at residential school for three years, he found out that he had a new baby brother at home in Eastmain. That was the good news. The bad news was that his mother had died the week after the baby was born. To make the bad news worse, Victor learned that he would not be allowed to go home to her funeral. Someone took him to his dorm, and he stayed there alone for a while, crying, and then they took him to someone's home in town. They brought his brother, who attended the other residential school in Fort George, to the same house and the two boys spent the day away from school, being together, comforting each other, and grieving their mom. The next day, they were back in their own schools again, like nothing had happened. Numbly, Victor finished out the school year and went home for the summer where he met his new baby brother.

The following school year, in November, back in residential school again, Victor got more bad news. At home in Eastmain, his nine-month-old baby brother had contracted pneumonia. It was fall, and the river was just starting to freeze: it was neither liquid enough for a seaplane to land safely nor frozen enough yet for a plane to use the ice as an airstrip. The swamp, where planes sometimes landed, was also not yet frozen enough. Eastmain had no other airstrip and no winter road to the South. There was no way to get his baby brother to a hospital. The baby died. Again, Victor and his brother were not permitted to attend the funeral.

The deaths separated Victor's family. Two sisters were adopted into other families, and his brother, another sister, and Victor stayed with their father and grandmother in Eastmain. For a few years then, from Grades Four to Six, Victor attended school in Eastmain and lived there year-round.

"You have to be able to look after yourself, Victor," his grandmother said. "You get only one life and you never know what's gonna happen. You have to know how to adapt."

She wanted him to be independent and self-sustaining. She wanted him to know how to cook and how to sew so that he could mend his own clothes if he needed to. She wanted him to learn everything he could, so that he could one day look after himself and be able to adapt to any situation. Eventually he used every skill he learned from her.

As for the stuff the priests had taught him, some of it, like French and English language studies, would eventually turn out to be useful. But some of it, like bead rituals and facing the right way during chapel and watching terrified kids on slippery poles, was pretty much useless.

Eventually, for Grades Seven to Ten, Victor was sent back to school on the island of Fort George. This time, though, things were different for Victor: for one, he was in the English sector instead of the French, and, more importantly, the Cree School Board had taken over the education system. The priests and counsellors with their strange and cruel ways were gone. There was no slapping, no force-feeding, no random punishments nor sudden torture. The bad stuff was gone. Victor lived with a Cree family who looked after him very well, and school was a very different experience from what it had been the last time he had lived in Fort George.

Around that time, the town of Fort George was being relocated to Chisasibi as part of the Hydroelectric Project. The relocation happened in the summer and, when Victor came back to school that September, he heard about how the buildings had been moved across the river on a barge. The white Roman Catholic church had been the biggest building to be moved and it had sat heavy on the barge, pushing down its enormous weight, greedy and oppressive. The barge had had to work harder for that church than for any other building, and the people watching could hardly see the barge itself. Even on the river, Victor thought, the church swallowed up so much more space than it should. Like the priests who had crushed the kids' language and beliefs, it seemed to drown everything but itself, and to rest on top of their grief like it was the only thing on the planet that mattered.

Victor finished high school there in the new location, one of the first students to graduate from the new school in Chisasibi.

At nineteen years of age, Victor boarded a bus headed for Montréal. It was dark when he stepped out of the Montréal bus terminal, and the city lights swamped him. The city was almost as bright at night as it would be in the daytime, and it was noisy and active and churning, like a big industrial machine at work. There was nothing sleepy or restful about it. *What have I got myself into*, Victor wondered. *What am I doing here?*

What he was doing was a 40-week auto mechanics course. It was quite an experience, studying like that in a college with people from all over the world, living in a culture that relied on gyms and swimming pools for fitness, instead of on water hauling and wood chopping and hunting, and that had restaurants on every street corner as if no one knew how to cook for themselves. The change was overwhelming, but Victor finished the course.

When he got back home to Eastmain, there wasn't much work for a mechanic, so Victor answered a posting for an observer-communicator at the airport. For training, Transport Canada flew him up to Fort Smith in the Northwest Territories, and, for a year and a half after that, he worked as an observer-communicator at the Eastmain airport. He made reports about weather, and spoke to the pilots over the radio as they flew in, telling them about wind speed and other things they needed to know to land safely. Then the Chief approached him, knowing he had taken an auto mechanics course, and asked if he was interested in studying to be a heavy machinery mechanic. It sounded interesting, so Victor flew back down to Montréal and took a 42-week heavy machinery mechanics course, came back to Eastmain, and started working as a heavy machinery mechanic.

Sometime around 2004, Victor was about 41 years old, and he went into the clinic for a routine check-up. The phone rang a week later calling him back in to speak to a nurse. When Victor walked into the nurse's office, she was already there. She held up two different bottles; they both held something that looked like blood, but one of them had a thicker consistency.

"This vial," she said, pointing to the first, "has regular healthy blood. This vial"—and she pointed to the second as if it repulsed her—"is your blood. It's not normal. You have diabetes." Her approach was harsh and aggressive and abrupt. The disease, she seemed to imply, was somehow his fault. He just wanted to leave the room and escape her aggression.

"Uh diabetes. Okay I'll, uh, I'll work on that," Victor said, and got out of there.

Later in the day, when he was on his way to work, the diagnosis sank in. He had diabetes. Well, that would explain why he had been so tired on the job lately. His co-workers had complained that he had even fallen fast asleep a few times. Victor laughed at himself then: he had thought that everyone was as sleepy on the job as he was and they had just been better at hiding it.

He didn't yet know very much about diabetes. He was supposed to take his pills, he knew, and at first he sometimes forgot, but soon they became part of his routine. He was sure of one thing, though: he would stay away from the clinic. He had had enough of being made to feel like something was wrong with him.

Around that time, the government announced it would launch inquiries into child abuse at residential schools. That same week, the mop-handle counsellor jumped off a bridge. So many kids had been hurt under his "guardianship." As far as Victor knew, none of them were the least bit unhappy about his suicide.

In 2010, Victor was at work. It was evening, and he was working alone, installing an injection pump into the engine of an excavator. Except for the noise of his tools, the big garage was quiet. He was standing on a platform, and there was a two-step screwed into the platform so it couldn't move. Victor moved to plug the hole where the timing bolt goes in, and the plug dropped to the floor. He turned around to step down—and lost his balance. He flailed and almost regained balance on the platform, but then fell to the floor four feet below. With the momentum of a 270-pound falling man, he hit the edge of a table on his way down.

Slowly, Victor got to his feet. He realized his head was bleeding so he went over the coffee break room to grab some napkins and soak up the blood. Then he called the clinic and told them he was hurt. Did he need an ambulance, they asked. No, he thought, he could get there himself.

At the clinic, they sewed seven stitches into the corner of his head where he had hit the table. Things were really starting to hurt. The following day, the clinic sent him to Chisasibi where they took x-rays, and from there, on the same day, they sent him to Amos to see another doctor for a full evaluation. After all the tests, Victor found out that, in addition to gashing his head, he had fractured his wrist, his elbow, and his kneecap. He went home with braces on his leg and wrist, and a sling for his elbow.

For a while, Victor couldn't go to work, but he could sit at home and think. Since his diabetes diagnosis, other than taking his pills, he hadn't really paid much attention to his health. Now, he had no choice but to think about it. *You get only one life,* he thought. *You have to be able to look after yourself.* He had a choice in front of him: he could either continue like this, ignoring his health for the most part and coping with the shakes and exhaustion that come with low and high blood sugar, or he could turn it around, adapt to diabetes like the fish had adapted to saltwater, and figure out how to be a healthy and agile adult.

Victor still didn't want to rely on the doctors and nurses at the clinic. He would keep up with regular check-ups, of course, but if he was going to get healthy, he would do it himself.

On November 4, 2012, still recovering from his injuries, he started on the treadmill. Just walking at first, for only five minutes.

Five minutes of walking was a very small thing to do, but he felt noticeably better. He did it almost every day until he was used to it. Then he walked for ten minutes. Then fifteen. After a while, he began to increase the speed of the treadmill until he was jogging for a few minutes. He kept at it until he could jog without stopping for 30 minutes. He started to include cycling then, just to see if he liked it. It was okay, so he kept it up and started to lift weights.

The numbers on the scale were going down, but what mattered more was that everything in his body began to work better. He slept more deeply at night and he moved more easily in the day. Some of the strength of his youth came back into his muscles, and the shakes came less frequently. And there were gadgets he could buy that made things kind of fun. He bought an app for his phone to keep track of his exercise. Seeing his progress charted on his phone was cool and undeniably satisfying.

Something about being fit made him want to change the way he ate. No way was he going to eat vegetables. Residential school, where he had been forced to eat vegetables after already having eaten a big meal, had made that pretty much impossible: any time he thought about eating vegetables, he always thought about things he didn't want to think about. But he could eat more fruit and more yogurt. He also didn't really want to eat junk food anymore, so he gradually cut out pop and chips. When he wanted a treat he reached for chocolate peanut butter cups—they were sweet, sure, but the peanut butter meant that his blood sugar didn't spike quite as badly as it did from other candy. Soon he felt like avoiding bread and eating less meat. And he even realized that he wanted to cut down on hard liquor; if he wanted alcohol, he reached for a beer instead, and not too much of that.

Even the smallest change made such a difference in the way he felt that he just wanted to keep at it. So he did something that many people have found impossible: after 32 years of smoking a pack a day, he smoked his last cigarette and quit, cold turkey. (Well, he tried nicotine patches for about twelve hours, but couldn't get them to stick.) He didn't smoke again after that.

One day, Victor realized he was probably going to live quite a bit longer than he would have, now that he had become a pretty healthy guy. He was fit, he had lost about a quarter of his body weight, he didn't smoke, and he took less diabetes medication than he had taken before. At this rate, he would probably be around to continue looking after his family in the way that his grandmother had looked after him. He had changed his life to take care of himself but it meant that he was taking care of his family and community too. It was a pretty good feeling.

The path had not been an easy. It had taken hard work and a good dose of commitment. And it had all started with a simple choice, a choice to be healthy. A choice that only he could make, that no one else could make for him.

Victor teaches his kids what his grandmother taught him. To be independent, to learn all kinds of skills, to take responsibility for their own health and well-being—and to be willing to adapt to a different way of living, a different kind of river water.

"You get one life," he tells them. "Make it count."

Stories We Heard Along the Way: Hunters

Most of the hunters in Eeyou Istchee grew up shooting geese and other small game with lead shot. Then Health Canada warned that lead shot could cause lead poisoning in the people who ate those geese. The hunters didn't want to make anyone sick and switched to steel shot. Steel shot, however, is a different weight than lead shot and it flies from the end of a barrel at a different velocity. Seasoned hunters who rarely missed their prey began to miss more often. Like kids with their first BB guns, they had to learn again how to shoot, and with time they got to know the weight and speed of steel shot and their aim once again became true.

•

There are many rules to respectful hunting and butchering and eating of bear. Certain parts of the bear must always be shared, and the skull should be nailed high on a tree out of respect for the animal. One of the most important rules is that the hunter must make eye contact with the bear before pulling the trigger. If a hunter has the bear in her or his sights but the bear doesn't meet the eyes of the person who will end its life, then the hunter must not pull the trigger. The bear lives for another day.

•

A culvert at the edge of the town of Nemaska is fed in part by a hot spring, and a small section of it never freezes over, not even in winter. A few years ago, a duck too wounded to fly south for the cold months stayed under the culvert in the warm section. The people in town knew about the duck and, even though it would have made a fine addition to any dinner table, no one shot it. The duck wintered there peacefully for several years.

•

A Cree hunter had been out on the land and was driving home along Route du Nord with a still-bloody moose carcass in the back of the truck. The weather was stormy and quite a bit of snow had already fallen when the truck hit an icy patch and overturned. Relatively unhurt, the hunter climbed out of his upside-down truck and hitched a ride into Mistissini with the next truck that came by. Soon a second truck came by and the people in it saw the overturned truck and blood everywhere. Panicked, they called the Nemaska ambulance and began to search through the snow for the bodies or wounded people who had lost all that blood. The ambulance arrived and the first responders poked long poles into the snow, especially in the bloodied areas, hoping for a soft and heavy hit that would indicate a body. Eventually they found the moose carcass and began to piece together what had happened. Not long after that, the driver returned with a tow truck, expecting to right his truck and pick up his moose. Instead he found an ambulance and a group of panicked people still looking for bodies.

•

A game warden pulled over a truck with several head of caribou in the back to check the hunters' licenses. The licenses were valid and it seemed like all was well until the warden, a hunter himself, noticed that the caribou on top poking out of the tarp looked a little odd, as if it hadn't been field-dressed in the usual way. He pulled back the tarp and began to examine the kill more thoroughly. The top caribou was completely unprocessed and had been carefully placed there to hide what was below: several baby caribou whose bellies had been opened, stuffed with cocaine, and then sewed shut. Their mouths had also been stuffed with cocaine. The warden figured that, even with climate change, cocaine had not become part of the caribou diet and he arrested the hunters.

8

The Story of Kimberly Coon of Mistissini

KIMBERLY watched the moose go down. From 200 metres away she could see that it was female. Her husband lowered the gun and they both headed through the woods, knives in hand. By the time they got to the animal, she had stopped breathing.

"Oh no," Kimberly said, "She's pregnant." The moose was even more magnificent close up, the size of her more imposing against brown shrubs and grasses.

"I know," her husband said. "It seems harsh. But it's the way of things. Our people have been doing this for centuries."

Kim nodded and knelt beside the moose and stroked the hide. She took a deep breath—and held it as her husband opened his knife and carefully sliced the belly. Hot blood and intestines spilled out steaming onto the spring snow. He sliced a bit further back and reached in and eased out the swollen uterus. He cut out the fetus, drained its blood, and wrapped it up. They turned to the adult moose then and separated out the intestines and organs, rinsed out the last of the blood, and field-dressed and sectioned it for transport. Then he walked back out to the truck and maneuvered it carefully through the woods as close as he could to the animal. Kim and her husband worked together then to load 1400 pounds of carcass onto the flatbed. Tonight, they would deliver the fetus to his parents (in Cree tradition, the choicest meats go to the elders), they would unload the carcass onto a layer of plastic on the spacious bathroom floor, and Kim would have a good sleep. She would carve it up in the morning.

She looked around once more before climbing into the truck for the drive home. She was always reluctant to leave the bush. Here, life was healthier, work stress and addictions less threatening, and her diabetes not nearly as bad. She brought her insulin along, of course; in town, she needed to inject it every time she ate. But in the bush, she needed it only at breakfast—when she ate toast and eggs, white foods, the foods of the colonizers. With the other meals, which were usually meat off the land, she rarely needed insulin. It wasn't just the food. In the bush, she had to collect and haul wood. She had to maintain a shelter. She had to build fires and cook over them and haul water to wash up after. If she didn't do these things, if she sat on her ass the way she did in her office at work, she wouldn't survive long. The exercise helped keep insulin levels steady and addictions at bay. She'd rather stay here.

She sucked in the clean air and let it out slowly. There was no going back. She lived in Mistissini. She was good at her job in the band office and she loved it. She had a beautiful red house with a spacious open kitchen and walls painted in warm orange tones. She had a bouncy one-eared dog out back and two healthy kids in her house and now her first grandchild crawled across the floors and laughed every time Kim came into the room. It was a good life. She couldn't not go back.

It hadn't always been a good life.

Kimberly's mother Louise had been an orphan. She was taken away from her only remaining family and sent to residential school in Ontario. She had enough to eat at school, she was not molested, and she was a good student who loved to study. But she was lonely, away from anyone she knew, and spent those years starved for attention and love. She found it with Kimberly's father, Simon. He had also gone through residential school but he had been badly treated. Together, the two of them worked hard and earned the respect of their peers and loved their kids, but they had lived intense and difficult lives and had developed addictions. Sometimes, at home, things got rough. On weekdays, Kim sat at the top of her class at school in Mistissini. But after school she went home to a life more complicated, a life of love and also of stress and addictions and anxiety.

Years passed, and Kimberly fell in love with a funny and shy man, Leonard, who reminded her of her dad and who came from a family that still practised traditional Cree ways. They were planning to spend winter in the bush that year. Kimberly was going along.

A winter in the bush meant weeks of prep work. They had to gather food supplies. They had to load up plywood and planks and canvas tarps to build a cabin and make the old outhouse snow-worthy again. They had to condition the chainsaws and generators and snowmobiles (there were no repair shops in the bush). They had to collect and prepare enough guns and ammunition for months of hunting everything from caribou to ptarmigan. They had to plan the hunts carefully so that there would be enough prey to hunt right to the end of winter. Kim had grown up an urban Cree and every bit of this process was new to her. Still, she did what she could to help (and felt a little embarrassed that she didn't know more).

Two weeks before they left, Kimberly and her boyfriend were drinking and got into a fight. For the first time ever, he beat her badly. The next day, she could hardly move. Angry welts streaked her arms and legs, her back and face. She had left her parents' house behind, but she had moved into another house where someone lived every day with an addiction. She had always thought that abused women should take their kids and leave their abusive homes. This was her chance, now that she wore the glossy bulbous bruises, to do just that—to leave her boyfriend and an addiction-centred life.

But what kind of choice *was* this? To stay and live with love and addictions and abuse, or to leave behind addictions and abuse but also love? There should be another way, she thought. She was smart. If she could just *manage* things properly, she might be able to make his addiction go away.

Kim did not leave Leonard. Two weeks later, she was in the bush with him and his family.

To start, they prepared the sturdy shelter for winter. It was a big job. Kim's task that first day was to shovel sand from a natural sandpit nearby into a pail, lug it back to the campsite, and pour it around the base of the shelter. The sand would help stabilize the shelter and seal the bottom from winter winds. Kim hauled and poured out the heavy sand. By noon, she didn't feel well, but kept working. Hour by hour, through the afternoon, she grew more nauseous. Sand is heavy, she was working hard, and she was still recovering from that beating. Was that all it was? Would it just pass?

Leonard's grandmother, who was preparing food for winter storage, watched her carefully all day long, worried. "Listen," she said to the others that evening. "I don't like the way Kim looks. I think she might be pregnant. I think she might be miscarrying right now. I think we have to get her to a hospital right away."

"We're out by Chisasibi!" someone said. "It's five hundred kilometres to a hospital! Isn't there a nurse around here?"

There was a hurried discussion—Kim was too sick by now to participate—and they decided not to question the old lady. Leonard's father helped Kim into the truck and drove her to the hospital that night, terrified to lose her and his grandchild. He drove faster than he had ever driven before, most of it over dirt roads that can quickly send a speeding truck into a spin. It was the scariest ride of Kimberly's life.

That was just the beginning of the drama.

Kim was in the hospital—and not in the bush—for a long while. There were tests, and more tests, and more tests still. She *was* pregnant and she *had* almost miscarried, Grandmother had been right. They barely saved the baby. Nearly every day of that pregnancy, Kimberly was sick with one thing or another. Then, after nine months of illness and a long labour, she wasn't able to birth the child naturally. The doctor had to do a last-minute C-section and surgically remove her daughter instead. The baby girl, at least, was healthy and beautiful.

And now there was another problem. The incision where the doctors had cut out the baby wasn't healing. It was oozing. Fluid and infection were building up painfully in Kim's abdomen. It got to be so bad that the doctor finally punctured the scar to make a hole for the fluid to drain out. Kim went home, all bandaged up, to rest.

There was no rest at home. Leonard never hit her again—but he was just 19 years old and not ready to stop partying. She spent the evenings in the house alone, trying to care for an infant and to recover from major surgery, and he spent them out, drinking. As much as she wanted to manage the situation, she couldn't do anything about his addiction if he wasn't there. And she was healing so badly that she could hardly manage herself and the baby. One night, she slid down to the floor and leaned back against the bed— just as the baby began to cry. Kim turned to get up. And realized too late that her muscles hadn't healed enough for her to get up from that position. No one was there to help her. She reached out to the bedside table, opened a drawer, and used it to hoist herself up. The whole process took seven minutes. The baby was okay when she finally got there, but what about the next time? So much could happen to a baby in seven minutes.

And that incision. Weeks had passed since the surgery and *still* it was oozing. Kim was at the clinic every single day. She was exhausted. She could see the worry on the nurse's face as he exchanged slimy dressings for fresh ones and took blood to test. It reminded Kim of the worry on Grandmother's face out in the bush. Finally, the doctor punctured the incision again and made a second drain for fluids to leave her body. A whole month later—with visits to the clinic every day to change the messy gauze dressings—the incision began to heal properly.

"Kimberly," the nurse said to her one day, "we have the results of your blood test now. I know why your incision isn't healing."

Kim looked at him sideways. She could feel more bad news coming on.

"You have diabetes," the nurse said. "Your pancreas isn't making insulin like it should, and your body needs insulin to fight infection and heal properly."

Kim looked down at the paper sheet that covered the bed she sat on. She knew the inside of this clinic better than she knew her own home.

"Diabetes?" she said, "What does that mean? I have to take some pills?"

"Ye—uh—it's a bit more involved than that."

Kim didn't really hear the rest of it. Some pills. She could take pills. Not a big deal. She had other things to manage.

With the proper meds, Kim's incision started to heal. But the diabetes and the pills were a big deal after all. She had to count out a specific number of pills before she ate, wait 30 minutes, and then eat a specific amount of food. If she ate more than the exact amount, her blood sugar would climb and she would be instantly exhausted, have trouble breathing, and feel horrible. If she ate less, her blood sugar would fall, her heart would race, she'd be weak, and would feel horrible. She couldn't eat chocolate cake, her favourite food in the world. She had to check the bottom of her feet every night for broken skin, and she had to be very careful any time she clipped her nails or scraped her skin. The tiniest cut had to be cleaned and treated right away or it became badly infected.

And, in truth, those pills *weren't* working well. They burned a hole right through Kim's stomach lining and she got an ulcer. More pills. The doctors switched the diabetes pills around and tried different combinations, but all of them caused problems. By the time her daughter was five years old, Kim didn't feel any less fragile than the day the baby had been cut out of her.

Before school one day, Kim chased her daughter around the house. They were both laughing hard. She leaned against a counter to catch her breath. This kid was amazing, Kim realized, the best part of her life. She wanted to be around to see her grow up and have kids of her own. With so many health problems, though, so many conditions and medications that weren't working in the ways they should—well, she might not live that long.

She was tired of being sick. She was tired of the drama.

Kim took her daughter to school as she had the day before and the day before that and went about her work the way she always had. But something had shifted. She didn't know how to go about it, but she knew she wanted to be healthier.

Getting healthy again, after so many years of illness and so many things she didn't understand, was not easy and it was not quick. There were two main health problems in her life—diabetes and addictions. Kim started with what she knew was good at. She was good at studying and she had plenty of willpower. She would learn what she could about diabetes.

One of the first things she found out was that exercise helped control the disease. She was too busy to go to the gym every day, so it would have to be walking. She walked with her daughter. She walked to the post office. Her house in Mistissini was about to be built, and she chose the site farthest away from her office so that she would be forced to walk one kilometre twice a day to and from work. Even on days she felt like being lazy, she found ways to move more.

And then there was food. Everyone knew that food affected diabetes—what she would do for a piece of chocolate cake again with a thick layer of frosting and maybe a sprinkle of coconut—but how, exactly? Kim spoke with diabetes experts and read everything she could find that talked about ingredients: pamphlets from the clinic, books, online articles. She had always felt better after a plate of whitefish or moose than after pizza or spaghetti, but she hadn't known that packaged and processed foods and anything made with flour made diabetes worse and traditional Cree foods did the opposite. She still had to eat processed foods sometimes—they were part of her life now—but whenever she could, she cooked things that didn't come in packages and she ate traditional fare.

It seemed that her own diabetes behaved differently than the diabetes described in the books. She did more research, this time about what the numbers on food labels meant and which ones affected diabetes. She began then to watch her blood sugar closely, pricking herself with a lancet, dripping blood on a strip, and pushing the strip into a glucometer many times a day. She copied down the numbers each time, and after a few weeks began to see patterns. At some times of day, her blood sugar was over 20, much too high, and at other times, it was too low. She looked for connections between her blood sugar numbers and the numbers on food labels and she adjusted what and how much she ate. Her fingers were numb from the pricking, but she was beginning to feel healthier.

Then she found out that she had misunderstood the insulin medication. She had believed that injecting insulin was only for people with serious diabetes, those almost dead. A nurse said, though, that insulin injections were especially good for anyone who needed flexibility. Her own pancreas had made insulin before she got diabetes. It was what her body wanted. It wouldn't burn her stomach, it wouldn't give her ulcers. No more taking pills and waiting thirty minutes before eating. With insulin, she could eat anything, even a slice of chocolate cake now and then, and inject the proper amount of insulin afterwards. Kim switched to insulin injections. The down side was—the needles. They were so long in those days that she had to lay the needle on the table and look at it for a while, psyching herself up before injecting. But her days got better and she felt so much healthier that the needles were totally worth it.

Kim was pregnant again. This time her boyfriend-who-was-now-her-husband was very supportive, and this time she didn't feel nauseous every day. This time, though, she had diabetes: if her blood sugar went too low, the baby's heart would be affected. With careful vigilance, Kim ate every four hours, even in the night, to protect the baby's heart. Those eight months were extremely stressful again, and she needed another C-section surgery one month early. Still, the baby was born with a healthy heart, and because Kim knew how to handle her diabetes, the incision healed faster.

In short, Kim would always have diabetes. It wasn't an enemy anymore. It was part of who she was, part of her life. She accepted it and worked to understand it and tried, as much as she could, to be healthy *with* diabetes.

Now she could turn her attention to addictions. Kim wasn't addicted to substances herself but her family had been shaped by drugs and alcohol abuse. With her diabetes, she had studied and then had done what she could. She would use the same method here, she thought, and help the people she loved. First, she joined the local Al-Anon, a group that supported people who lived with addicts. They had just a few people, and they, like Kim, had all been deeply affected by addictions. Slowly, to this comfortable group, she began to talk about substance abuse. Addiction was not something to be ashamed of, they said, but a disease. She should speak of it openly and honestly and—especially important—without judgment.

This was a new way of thinking. She had been surrounded by addicts her whole life, but there was plenty about addiction she didn't know. Someone told her about a college in North Bay with a program in Addictions Prevention. Kim was looking for a change. She moved to North Bay and enrolled. She would study to become an addictions counsellor.

Kim got the surprise of her life. The first thing she learned at college was that she was an addict after all. Her need for control didn't come in a bottle or a packet, but it was a serious addiction of its own. She was what they called an *addiction enabler*: she tried to control the addicts in her life by helping them too much. When her husband had been drinking and was unable to work, for instance, she would call in sick for him. She had thought that if she could just do enough to keep his life stress-free, he would stop drinking too much. She had thought she was being supportive. Her sacrifices, though, had made it *easier* for him to be addicted. She had worn out the people around her with her need for control and her desire to fix things—and, with all that stress, she had worn herself out too. (Stress, the doctor said, made diabetes worse.)

Then a second surprise: she would never be able to fix any-one's addiction—snap—just like that, not even her own. Recovery was a lifelong process, and, like diabetes, it had to be integrated into everyday life. The addict had to make one healthy choice, and then make another one, and then make another one, for the rest of her life. Like every other person, she would have to make her own life. Surrounded by positive, cheerful people at her school and by more support than she had ever had, Kim began her long recovery from addiction.

It wasn't easy. Every time Kim wanted to fix someone else's problem, she wrote in her journal and tried to understand why she felt that way. She worked hard to focus on accepting the addictions in herself and her family instead of being angry about them or trying to cover things up. It was not her job to make other people sober, but it was her job to build honest and compassionate relationships free from judgment and shame. Soon after Kim stopped enabling, her husband stopped drinking altogether. His addiction was not her fault nor her responsibility. But it became easier for him to recover when she was not enabling.

Kim was back in her bathroom in the warm red house, kneeling on the floor. It was time to carve up the moose carcass spread out on plastic in front of her. They would need the meat for her granddaughter's walking-out feast in a few months. Years ago, young urban Kim wouldn't have known where to start, but she had been learning the traditional ways for a while now, and carving the moose came more naturally. Kim could hear her son playing on his gaming console, and her daughter, now 17, playing in the living room with *her* baby daughter. Her daughter and the baby would be moving to North Bay next year for college. Kim knew she would miss them terribly.

She had taken the week off of work to volunteer in National Addictions Awareness Week. The old ones, the traditional Cree, had understood the importance of integration. Their spirituality, which was more important to Kim now than it had ever been, emphasized balance in the four directions—of the spirit, the physical body, the emotions, and the intellect. Colonization, the coming of the white people, had brought about imbalances and a massive increase in diabetes and addictions in Cree communities. This long-ago event had really affected Kim's life. She couldn't go back in time. The white people and their ways were here now and, like diabetes and addictions, they had to be integrated into life.

There were still difficult days. Kim still had plenty of stress and she wasn't quite on top of her diabetes. There were more changes to make. But it had become a good life, one day at a time.

9

The Story of James Jonah of Waskaganish

AFTER thinking about it for a long time, James Allan Jonah came to understand a few things about health in Eeyou Istchee and its history of colonization.

Many years ago, before the white people colonized this land, the people of the Cree Nations could eat any food the Creator had given them, as long as it hadn't spoiled, without getting sick. They could eat moose or fish or partridge until they were full and it was nutritious and their blood sugar levels remained balanced and healthy. The food itself was satisfying and small portions were enough to get people through a whole day's work without craving more—and that was important because the food had to be portioned out to last until the next hunt or until the end of winter. It was the same with the medicine the Creator had provided. Traditional remedies were safe and effective. If someone accidentally swallowed too big a dose of beaver musk tea or applied twice as much tree sap as needed to a wound, they would not be poisoned. The body would take in the medicine and heal, and the people didn't have to worry about toxic side effects.

When the white people came, they brought a different way of eating, a different kind of food, and a different kind of medicine.

They depended on the clock and ate at regular times of day, whether or not they were hungry. Their food was processed; the grains had been ground into flour, their fruit and cane had been powdered into intensely sweet concentrates, their breads and cereals had been laced with chemical preservatives. In smaller portions, the processed food could be tolerated. But if the people ate too much flour or sugar at one sitting, they would throw up or fall asleep, and if they ate too much of it every day, their organs would be taxed to the point of eventually shutting down. Their medicines were dangerous too: nearly all of them were poisonous in large doses and many of them came with serious side effects. At times the medicines caused problems worse than the illnesses they were meant to treat.

The white people told their children stories of villains and heroes being changed by a single bite of something so they would know the dangers of their food and medicines. They told of a mushroom that would make a girl grow bigger than a house,[1] of fruit coated with a drug and one bite would drop a grown woman into a coma,[2] of gingerbread walls that lured children to a person who wanted to eat them,[3] and of a sweet that drove a boy so mad with cravings he betrayed his nation for another mouthful.[4]

The old Cree didn't tell the same stories to their children. Their stories talked about animals providing food, so when you ate you took in the animal spirits. Eating was part of a spiritual connection to the land and food should be treated with reverence and respect. They had never heard of food that produced cravings yet didn't satisfy hunger, or of medicine that made people sick. Surely such food wouldn't be called food, and such medicine wouldn't be called medicine. When the white people set their food and medicine in front of the people of the Cree nation, they didn't

1. *Alice in Wonderland* by Lewis Carroll.
2. "Snow White and the Seven Dwarves."
3. "Hansel and Gretel."
4. *The Lion, the Witch, and the Wardrobe* by CS Lewis.

talk about cravings or about the dangers of overeating processed foods, and they didn't say anything about their medicines having side effects that could hurt them badly.

In Eeyou Istchee, there are stories of the arrival of ice cream. Of Cree people who had never eaten something so sweet, who sat down and ate a whole four-litre bucket without stopping. And then going to the store to buy another bucket. They thought it was food. They thought it was healthy and nutritious, like the sweet berries they ate in summer. And they couldn't stop eating it.

Some elders were suspicious. Food shouldn't affect people like that, they thought. It should satisfy hunger; it should never compel people to eat more and more, and it should never consume the mind with cravings.

"Don't eat it," they said to their friends. "It will hurt us all eventually."

But many people were addicted after the first bite, and, like the boy in the white-culture story who had eaten the wrong sweet, they were so fixed on their craving for another bite that they couldn't hear the people who knew processed food was bad for them.

James Allan Jonah had his first mouthful of ice cream when he was eight years old. After that first taste, ice cream was always on his mind. When he looked up at the sky or down at the snow, he thought about ice cream because he thought clouds and snow both looked like ice cream. If you had seen him walking to school or swimming with his friends and you had asked him what he was thinking about at that very moment, he would have said, "Ice cream, of course."

But in those days ice cream was hard to come by. There were no refrigerated trucks transporting frozen foods all the way north to Waskaganish. In summertime, anything coming into town was on the slow, unrefrigerated barge. For ice cream, James had to wait for winter when it could stay frozen on the Austin Airways plane all through the long trip north. The first snowfall of late October or early November always filled James with joy: soon, very soon, it would be cold enough for ice cream.

In the next few years, James tasted other processed foods like hamburgers and macaroni and white rice. He learned quickly how to prepare them, and, because he craved them constantly, they became his everyday foods, followed by desserts of canned peaches or frosted cakes or chocolate bars. From his parents' teachings, he knew the spiritual significance of food, and so James prayed over his hamburgers and rice and peaches. As long as he did that, he thought, he was taking in the necessary spiritual components, respecting the land and the animals, and continuing the spiritual ways of the Cree.

James's father was one of those suspicious of processed foods. He continued to hunt and fish and to eat traditional foods—moose and fish and beaver fat, goose and grouse and bear fat. Sometimes he spread crushed fish that had been mixed with goose grease onto bannock—which was made from processed flour—but most other white-culture foods he didn't touch.

He looked at James's plate with concern.

"Son," he said, "there's something wrong with that food. I can't tell you what it is, but I worry it'll kill you."

Around that time, James heard about diabetes for the first time. It was a disease, he knew, that made people very sick. Anyone who had it, he thought, would slowly begin to die. One by one their organs would shut down and their limbs would get infected and have to be amputated. He didn't know then that the way he was eating was already taxing his pancreas and kidneys, and already putting him at risk for diabetes.

Many years later, when he was 38 years old, he was diagnosed with diabetes. Terrified by thoughts of organ malfunction and limb amputation, he got very upset. He didn't believe it was true. He refused to take medication for it. He cried, and then, slowly, he slumped into a deep depression.

At the age of 40, James had an unforgettable dream. He stood outside in a natural meadow. All the colours were saturated— the sky an intense robin-egg blue, the grass shining yellow from the light of the sun, and the trees the richest jewel green he had ever seen. For a while, he stood there in the meadow, taking it all in. Then an enormous eagle flew out of the forest right towards him. Peace flooded over James. It was the most elegant animal, its flight confident and effortless as if it simply rested on wind thermals. James felt connected to the eagle. It circled over him and returned to the forest. And then, as if it had changed its mind, the eagle flew towards James again, this time much lower. It passed over his head and James could see individual fibres in the feathers and the curl of the talons. The wind generated by the massive wings cooled his face.

Three days later, while James was at work, he felt a pinch in his chest that grew deeper until he had a hard time breathing and fell on the floor. He was having a heart attack.

The eagle predicted this, he thought, *when it came for me in my dream.*

His coworkers rushed him to the clinic where doctors put him on a plane and airlifted him to Montréal. On the plane, he had a second heard attack.

The eagle predicted this too, James thought, *when it came around a second time.*

His cholesterol was so high, the doctors said, that plaques in his blood had blocked an artery and had twice stopped the flow of blood to his heart. Like diabetes, high cholesterol could sometimes be genetic, they said, and, like diabetes, it could sometimes come from eating too much of the wrong foods.

James recovered slowly.

He had survived, but what a wake-up call. If he wanted to live a full life, he was going to have to take his cholesterol and diabetes more seriously. And, at over 400 pounds, he was going to have to start by thinking differently about food. Thinking about food took his mind to a nice big bowl of chocolate ripple ice cream with hot fudge sauce and roasted almonds. He imagined the taste of it, the smoothness coating his tongue and sliding down his throat. Already he craved it.

He knew then—this was going to be a difficult path to walk.

Medication quickly brought James's cholesterol to healthier levels, and then the doctors put him on insulin to control his diabetes. The cholesterol medication didn't bother him, but James felt the insulin affecting his circulation. His hands and feet would grow cold and numb, something he had never experienced before. And his appetite became so uncontrollable that he quickly gained 40 lbs.

"I have to stop using this," he said to his doctor. "I have to bring my eating and diabetes under control another way."

He stopped taking the insulin and began overhauling his food habits instead. He wrote a long list of changes he would have to make to his diet. No cookies, no fries, no cheeseburgers, no McDonalds, no pop, no chips, no Tim Hortons, no doughnuts, no cakes, no canned peaches, no toast, no cheesecake, no poutine, no rice, no cereal, and, grievously, no ice cream. Every single one of them was addictive to him. No sooner would he decide to give something up than he would crave it with every cell in his body. He could hardly do his work for the longing. He even had to stop chewing gum: it didn't worsen his diabetes or cholesterol, but the little taste of sugar in his mouth brought about intense cravings for more. Quitting each processed food was an extended battle of will that did not get easier with time. Every day, James woke up thinking about sugar.

No longer eating the very foods he had relied upon for decades seemed so unnatural. Sometimes James thought he couldn't continue this path. He would slump again into a depression and be unable to get out of bed. Or he would relapse and begin again to eat sugar—and immediately get sick. He would flip on the television to distract himself from cravings with a cop show or *National Geographic* documentary, only to be assaulted with commercials about milkshakes or cheesecake or chocolate bars. He would pick up a book to read about something other than food—and someone in his family would plunk down beside him and with a bowl of ice cream or a bag of chips, and James could hardly turn the page for longing. People who weren't diabetic or who had never been addicted to processed foods didn't understand how difficult every day was. Sometimes James's frustration was so intense that he wondered if his family even wanted him around.

Thankfully, he had traditional foods. If he ate some fish or moose or beaver or grouse, even in small amounts, his hunger would be sated. He might still crave sweets or chips, but at least he would not be hungry. The thing is, traditional foods were not easy. The animals had to be hunted and killed, then field dressed and transported back to town, the skin or scales had to be removed, they had to be butchered or filleted or smoked, and the cooking inevitably took a long time. Another problem was that so many people in his community liked to prepare hunted game with barbecue sauce or with ketchup and mustard—which were all loaded with sugar and preservatives. One small taste of that sauce, and the craving for more, for sugar, took over James's brain. And so he would eat his traditional food without sauce and try not to think about what the others at the table were eating or how alone diabetes made him feel.

That was how James learned about the dangers of processed foods.

Without a doubt, the changes James made were helping. In time—a few years—he felt healthier. He slept better, he could move more easily, his heart felt stronger, his thirst and weariness had disappeared. And, as an added bonus, over a hundred pounds had

slowly melted away. Every now and again, he ate something processed, a doughnut or a small bowl of ice cream, but it was a treat,
something rare that helped him not to feel deprived, and he was
careful not to make it a habit.

Unfortunately, the changes were still not enough and he had
to take pills to control his blood sugar levels. Soon it became clear
that the pills had little effect on James, so the doctor prescribed a
different diabetes pill instead.

A few days after James began to take the new pill, he felt
horrible. His hips and knees and elbows ached. His leg muscles
cramped violently, his feet throbbed whether or not he walked
on them, and his abdomen hurt constantly, deep in the organs
and through to his back. What was going on now, he wondered.
Had he developed a cancer? One day, when he was driving to
Waskaganish from Val-d'Or, it was so bad that he couldn't even
make the drive. He had to stop half way in Washaw Sibi for the
night, just to rest.

While he was there, a friend who had been a nurse's aide for
many years eyed him with concern. "Can I see your medication?"
she asked.

James passed her the bottle of pills, wiped sweat from his
brow, and curled into a ball around his hurting stomach.

"These pills are probably causing all that pain," she said. "You
might have pancreatitis or kidney problems from the medication.
When you get home, go on the internet and read about this medication and the side effects."

James looked at her in disbelief, and the next day, when
he got home, he did exactly that. Some people experienced side
effects from this pill, the medical website said, and the side effects—
his symptoms exactly—could put him on dialysis for the rest of his
life or even kill him. Immediately he stopped taking the medication,
and in a few days all the pain and all the cramps were gone.

James was upset. He paid the doctor another visit.

"Why didn't you tell me that this medication had these horrible side effects? Why didn't you tell me that these pills could hurt me?"

"The side effects don't happen to everyone," the doctor said. "If I had told you about them, you might have convinced yourself that you were having the side effects even if you weren't."

"But even if I believed the pills were helping me," James said, "they still would actually be hurting me! Even if they were managing my diabetes, they might be killing me in some other way! And you're prescribing this to people who might not understand how to go online to learn about it, or might not even realize they are feeling sick from their medication instead of their diabetes! People who won't question you because their cultural norms see that as disrespectful, or people who can't defend themselves against you! Why don't you at least *tell* people about the drugs you prescribe? Or give them a list of side effects to watch out for??"

James was so upset he didn't even listen to the doctor's answer and walked out.

And that was how James learned about the dangers of Western medicine.

After thinking about it for a long time, James would like to see some changes in the ways the James Bay Cree deal with illness and health. First, he would like to see every Cree person who takes medication find out everything they can about the medicine they take. How does it work in the body? How might it affect someone in the short term? In the long term? How soon should they expect to feel differently? What are the common and uncommon side effects that patients should look out for when they take it? Even if they don't experience side effects, James thinks they should still understand the medication they take. The doctors don't always tell their patients about medicines and side effects, and people in Eeyou Istchee often don't receive the printed information about medications that patients are given in the South, so people taking medication should be prepared to do their own research. James would like to see the Cree Board of Health organize a way to make drug information available even to people who don't know how to use computers or libraries: plain-language or Cree-language information sheets might work or conversations that patients can have with someone who understands medication and who speaks Cree.

Second, he would like to see the James Bay Cree and their doctors find ways to develop relationships of mutual respect. In many cases, respect is already there and most Cree people, including James, are grateful for the doctors. But every now and again, James hears about another Cree person and another and yet another who feels like he is being experimented upon with medication as if he were a lab rat or not listened to as if she were a stump or a stone. These patients begin to think of their doctors as drug dealers who prescribe without considering the person in front of them, and no longer see them as healers. They lose confidence in doctors and even suspect them of misinforming patients or withholding information just to get someone out of the office. Some patients become so suspicious of medication that they stop taking it even if it's keeping them alive and so afraid of doctors that they don't visit the clinic even when they are very sick. These relationships are the ones James would like to see repaired.

Third, he would like to see a region-wide diabetes support group built with the support of the Cree Government. Right now, diabetes is one of the biggest crises facing the Cree nation, and it seems to James that many people aren't taking it seriously. He sees people with diabetes depend on medication without ever hearing that other methods of diabetes management exist, methods like the food control that James chose, or exercise or stress management. Of course, people with diabetes might choose not to try these other methods of managing diabetes—they can be difficult—but at least they should know about them. If the alternate methods were talked about in a support group across Eeyou Istchee, they would soon be common knowledge. And a support group could go a long way to helping people with diabetes feel included rather than excluded: not only could they meet others with the same disease and feel less alone, they could also bring family members who might learn from the group how very difficult it can be to live with diabetes.

Fourth, James would like to see more naturopathic medicine come into the Cree way of healing. The old Cree had traditional medicines to treat all kinds of illnesses and the stories show they had a high rate of success. But today, when people get sick, they most often visit the clinic for Western medication instead of visiting an expert in traditional medicines. Beautiful Western clinics have been built in each community and fundraising has been done for expensive dialysis machines in those communities that don't already have them. James would like to see traditional medicine pharmacies and practitioners brought into each community too so Cree traditional healing could be offered alongside the Western methods used in the clinics. He'd also like to see natural medicine conferences in Eeyou Istchee every year or two, with speakers who are experts in systems of healing from around the world: Chinese acupuncture, for instance, which is thousands of years older than Western medicine, or Reiki and other methods of energy healing, or traditional herbal medicine systems from across the globe. With all the money going to clinics and doctors and pharmacies and dialysis, James thinks that surely a small amount can be directed towards exploring additional ways of doing medicine.

The people of Eeyou Istchee have been struggling with Western food and medicine for a long time, and the numbers of the sick and dying are only getting higher. Maybe it's time to do something different about it. Maybe it's time to bring in more options.

10

The Story of Martha Sheshamush
of Whapmagoostui

INSIDE the teepee, young Martha watched her mother take the beaver from her father. Instantly his muscles relaxed and his back straightened—it was a heavy animal, about forty pounds, and he had brought it all the way back to the camp carefully so as not to damage the fur. He went back outside as her mother laid the beaver on its back, took up her knife, and began to cut. The musk and castor glands had already been removed, so she slit the lustrous pelt up the belly to the mouth, she used a bone tool to separate skin from flesh, she severed the paws at the first joint, she opened the belly and gutted it, and she sliced off the tail. Every part of the animal would be used, nothing wasted. Then she built up the fire and soon the camp smelled of roasting beaver.

There would still be enough beaver meat for another day or two, but Martha knew her father would rise early the next morning, while the light was still grey, and set out again for a day of hunting or fishing, and her mother would be ready to process the kill. It was hard work to feed a family on the land.

Times change. Martha's family moved into town where her parents found jobs. Before, they had lived in the bush eight months a year. But life in town was expensive. Rent to pay, groceries to buy. Now they could take just one month away from their work to be in the bush.

Martha hated town life. The food was *so bad*. People opened boxes and ate the stuff inside. They dumped cow milk over cardboard flakes and called it cereal; Martha called it "Sawdust After a Hard Rain." Their "bread," made of flour, was already dry as dust and they toasted it so that it was drier still and impossible to swallow. They ate things that came wrapped in plastic or that had corners. What kind of food had *corners*? But what could she do? She was a kid. She couldn't just walk back out into the bush by herself. Martha didn't get used to town food for a long time.

She could see that her dad wasn't excited about town life either. In the bush, he had to work, dawn to dusk, just to hunt enough food and chop enough wood to keep his family alive. He was always busy doing something and it was always essential to their survival. In town, he got behind the wheel of his truck, drove to the store, and bought what he needed and carried it home in a bag. The boredom, the unimportance of it, lay plain on his face. From time to time, he would drink with his so-called friends in town. It didn't mean anything—it was just what people in town did to fill the time.

Until she finished elementary school, Martha stayed in the Whapmagoostui town with her family, longing for the bush. And one day she didn't miss the bush anymore. She had become used to living in town.

In those days, Whapmagoostui had no high school, and, when Martha reached high school age, she was sent to Chisasibi, a town 200 kilometres further south. There, she lived with her grand-mother and attended high school classes.

Martha hated it. Oh, the people were nice enough, she loved her grandmother, and the class material was interesting, but every house, every snowfall, every person she saw made her homesick. She wanted to be home with her family, either in Whapmagoostui or out in the bush, it didn't matter. Just not in Chisasibi.

So, over the next year, Martha learned the correct answers to the material taught in class—and, methodically and deliberately, she wrote the *incorrect* answers in every test she took. In Math class, in French class, in History class. She failed Grade 9 and failed it spectacularly. A complete triumph. Anyone who assigned as many tests and exams as these school people did, she thought, would not take well to such failure. Surely they would give up on her now and send her home where she could live with her family. Surely, she had changed her life.

Unfortunately, the school people didn't give up that easily. They just made her repeat Grade 9. The whole year, all over again.

Martha didn't give up either. Throughout the second year of Grade 9, once again, she filled in the wrong answers (though she knew the right ones), and waited to be sent home.

They just made her repeat Grade 9 a third time. And after that they sent her even farther south, all the way down to Val-d'Or, for Grades 10 and 11.

Martha stopped trying to fail. It didn't work anyways. She was just getting farther and farther from where she wanted to be. Instead, she gave them what they wanted in her courses during the week—and drank with her friends every weekend. It didn't mean anything. It was just what you did to pass the time in small-town Val-d'Or. Eventually, it became a normal thing to have a drink or two on weekdays too. Then it became normal to drink more than two drinks and to drink every day.

Somewhere in there, Martha got used to being in school away from her family.

So she kept going to school, even after High School, and

finished a Bachelor's Degree in Social Work at the University of Québec. Later, she went to North Bay for more schooling and got a Diploma in Mental Health and Addictions and studied, for the first time, Indigenous Studies and the history of her own people and their move from the bush into settlements.

After university, Martha finally returned to Whapmagoostui, where she got married and had kids. She had been drinking for a while now but her kids were pretty great. Once she had them, she didn't want to drink because it wasn't good for them. She wrestled the addiction for a couple of years until she was able to stop altogether.

Fifteen years passed and it was 2010. Martha lay in the hospital bed in Val-d'Or. A glass of stale water and a plate of cold food sat neglected on the mobile tray. She felt awful. She had felt awful before—try moving from the bush into town, or leaving your family for high school, or birthing kids—but this was worse. This time she felt mutilated. She wasn't herself anymore. The surgeon had chopped out her uterus and she couldn't have more kids. She lifted her gown and looked at the dressing covering the wound. Blood and pus were oozing onto the gauze. She lowered the gown again, pushed the mobile tray down to the end of the bed, gingerly lay back, and went back to sleep.

There had been some complications in the surgery. For a full week, Martha lay in a hospital bed, watching the hospital TV. Then she went home, but there, too, she lay on the sofa and watched TV. She was still too sick to be up and doing things around the house, and she was much too sick to go back to work. Martha healed, but slowly, slowly. When she was frustrated that she couldn't move more easily, she reached for a bag of chocolate chips. When she was overcome with sadness at not being able to have more children, she reached for potato chips. And when she was upset over all the parts of her life that someone else had chosen, someone else had controlled, she reached for Oreo cookies and licked out the filling first. The junk food was comforting, a reliable old friend. It never sent her away, and it never cut her up.

After three months of eating and no exercise and a slow, painful recovery, Martha could move more easily again, but she had gained 60 lbs. She had gained so much weight so quickly that people who hadn't seen her in a while asked if she was pregnant.

She would much rather have been pregnant.

Two and a half years later, in 2013, the old surgery complications were still bothering her. She hadn't been feeling like herself. She wasn't interested in anything, she had never cared less about things that were supposed to matter, and when she sat down to type at work, her hands shook so badly that she hit the wrong keys. Her old Social Work and Mental Health textbooks talked about depression—maybe that's what she had. Martha went to the clinic. The doctor would probably run tests and send her home with some SSRIs, that medication they gave people nowadays for depression.

Sure enough, the doctor did run the routine tests, and he did send her home with medicine but it was medicine for diabetes. Her blood sugar levels were so high there could be no doubt that her pancreas had stopped working properly and she had diabetes.

Martha went home, threw the pamphlets in the garbage, and plopped onto the sofa. She needed to wallow. She knew about diabetes. She knew people who had it. She knew exactly what was in front of her. When she had been younger, she had always been thin and had been sure she would never be one of those diabetics. And now, probably because of that stupid surgery—that mutilation— and difficult recovery after, here she was, with this stupid disease.

The times had changed again.

Diabetes. Martha hated it. The pills made her feel *off*. Sure there were people who could control their disease just by eating carefully and exercising regularly. It would be great to be one of them. But that was a faraway goal to reach and, in all honesty, she had no motivation. She could hardly force herself even to make the small changes from junk food to healthier snacks, let alone the big shifts she would have to make in eating, in exercise, in stress management to get off the pills. She didn't want to be here, in this situation, this woman with diabetes who now was supposed to overhaul her life. She hadn't chosen this.

Martha thought back to her grandmother who had had diabetes too. Martha remembered her opening tins of tomato soup or cooking noodles. She had always cared about her diet, about eating well, but she would not have known about the hidden sugars in those foods. That they would have made her feel worse.

Day after day, as Martha counted out her pills, she began to think about the bush. Moving back to the bush, now, years after she had left it, would be the easiest, most satisfying way to take control of the situation. Her parents had moved back onto the land when her mom retired. One of her sons had moved out there too, years ago, wanting to live in the traditional ways. There were no chips to reach for when things got stressful and, anyways, things didn't get very stressful in the bush. It was peaceful. You didn't have to think about exercise or going to the gym: you hunted animals, you maintained cabins, you chopped wood, you prepared food, you *moved.* All day long.

She and her husband could quit their jobs, couldn't they? You don't need money in the bush, her father had taught her that. Even thinking about the bush made her feel better. The problem was the four dead-of-winter months when you *had* to live in town, when hardly anyone stayed in the bush anymore. How could they pay for those four months if they quit their jobs? Could they figure something out? Maybe, eventually.

In the meantime, Martha was at home, on her sofa, and— she groaned out loud the moment she realized this—it was going to have to be the gym. A few years back she had taken BounceFit classes. Once she had started going, it had been easy to keep going, they had been so much fun. These days her friends took Boot Camp classes. They would welcome her, of course. But those first few classes—ugh! Her legs would burn and her muscles would shudder and each one-hour class would feel like it was seven hours long. She could hardly face that again.

There was her son, packing his shoes and gloves for weight-lifting at the gym. And her husband rustling through the closet for his bag of exercise gear to go along. His blood sugar levelled right out after each exercise session, she knew, and it shot right back up if he took a few days off of exercising. A blast of cool air as the door closed behind them.

Stupid diabetes. The next time the boys went to the stupid gym, she was going to have to go too. She was going to hate it, she already knew.

And a couple of weeks later, in Boot Camp with her friends, she was already used to it. It wasn't so bad.

Stories We Heard Along the Way: Government

After years of court battles, the James Bay Northern Quebec Agreement was finally drawn up. The Grand Chief of Eeyou Istchee and the nine chiefs of individual communities neatly signed their names to the paper, each on the line provided for him. Québec premier Robert Bourassa, though, was perhaps feeling a little insecure that day: like the scrawl of a child, his signature is so huge that it takes up nearly a third of the page.

•

There was a contest once, a game among friends, about who could tell the biggest lie. The prize went to the fellow who said this: "I'm from Indian Affairs. I'm here to help."

•

For a few winter seasons, the government people dropped off food that they considered appropriate for winter in Eeyou Istchee: canned tomatoes, boxes of dried macaroni, and a pale orange processed-cheese product called Velveeta. The people boiled them up together in big pots and that's how they got the recipe for Government Soup.

•

A few years ago, as part of the Canada-wide *Idle No More* movement, David Kawapit, a young man from Whapmagoostui (our northern-most community), decided to take on a traditional long-distance journey of unity and walk/snowshoe to Ottawa to speak with former Prime Minister Stephen Harper about various Indigenous concerns. He, along with Stanley George, Travis George, Johnny Abraham, Raymond Kawapit, Geordie Rupert, and guide Isaac Kawapit, left on

16 January 2013, in the dead of winter, in temperatures of below minus 40 degrees, pulling their supplies behind them. They snow-shoed and showshoed and walked and walked, sometimes hunting for food along the way, sometimes sleeping out of doors, sometimes resting in communities. They travelled 1600 kilometres, they carried a unity stick, and they followed traditional trade routes of the Algonquin, Mohawk, and Cree. From time to time, others would join and walk part of the way with them. Word spread about the Journey of Nishiiyuu, as it came to be called, and by the time they reached Ottawa, nearly 400 people were walking alongside. They walked along Ottawa streets, to Victoria Island (a traditional Algonquin meeting place where three rivers converge), and approached Parliament Hill to address Mr. Harper. Thousands of people greeted them at Parliament Hill. Mr. Harper, having heard that David and the Nishiiyuu walkers would arrive that day, chose not to meet them and instead visited the panda bears at the Toronto Zoo. Panda diplomacy, evidently, was a higher priority for him than First Nations-Government of Canada relations. Isaac Kawapit, the guide, passed away a few months after the walk was completed.

•

Years ago, the Indigenous people of Canada were forbidden by the government to drink alcohol. Every now and then, an RCMP representative would travel through looking for moonshine even though it was obvious there was none there. He would go through the camp nevertheless and tear everything up, destroy things, and make a huge mess. Then he'd leave.

11

The Story of Emily Wesley of Oujé-Bougoumou

YOUNG Emily Wesley lived with her mother in Moosonee. Every day before school and again after dinner, Emily brought her mother a pin. Her mother pricked one of her own fingers and squeezed a drop of blood onto a piece of paper. She slotted the paper into a machine and a number showed up on a computer monitor. Emily's mother read it and told Emily how much medication she needed. Emily filled a big metal needle with the right amount and gave it to her. As she watched, her mother lifted her shirt and stuck the needle into her stomach. After she had finished, Emily carried the used needle into the kitchen where she washed and sterilized it in boiling water, along with the empty bottle from her mom's medicine, and put them both away. At the end of the day, just before bed, Emily's mother took off her socks and Emily looked carefully over every inch of her mom's feet and toes. Emily's grandfather had the same diabetes disease that her mother had, but he had had it for much longer—and it had cost him both legs. A small cut on his foot had once become infected and hadn't been able to heal, and eventually the infection had spread until the leg had to be cut right off. First one leg and then the other. Emily wanted her mom to live a long life with both of her legs, so if she saw even a tiny scratch or crack she would clean and treat and moisturize it right away.

Over time, even with Emily and her mom doing everything they knew how to do to keep her mom healthy, her mother got sicker. She lost her eyesight, she got heart disease, and eventually her kidneys began to falter and she needed home dialysis.

Once, Emily saw her mother move slowly to the table and sit down and write a letter. She was writing to Emily's father who lived in Québec. Emily knew what the letter said. It said this: "Your daughter Emily is a smart and beautiful girl. She helps me every day. Come and visit her so that she can know her father."

He never did. Emily grew up without meeting her dad. He was killed in a car accident in 1980.

After she finished high school, Emily decided to go to school and be a nurse. But the band in Moosonee, where she had grown up, was bankrupt and had no money to pay for her schooling.

"It's time you meet your father's family anyways," her mom said. "Let's visit them in Waswanipi. If it's okay there, maybe you can stay, and maybe his band will have money to pay for your school. I'll come back and manage here. We'll talk every day on the phone."

So they packed their bags with everything they needed for a few days, including her mother's medications, and they went to Waswanipi, Eeyou Istchee, and met her dad's family. Emily could see that her mom was so happy to introduce her daughter to them, so happy they could all spend some time together, even if it was just for a few days.

At one point, they were visiting someone in town and there was a noise at the door. A person was pushing through, saying "Where is she? Where is she?" A big man wrapped Emily up in his arms in one big overpowering hug and he didn't let go for a long time. "I'm so glad you're here, I'm so glad you're here," he said, over and over, and cried. He was her uncle, her father's brother, he finally said when he stopped squeezing her, and he was so grateful for Emily in his life to remind him of his brother. It lessened the pain of his loss.

Her mom went back home and left Emily alone with her father's family. It was a strange time. Emily's dad had been gone for six years already and now his friends said that he had talked about her, about a daughter who lived far away in Moosonee, but he hadn't given them details. *What details could he give?* she thought. *He knew almost nothing about me. He never bothered even to visit me. He wouldn't have recognized me if he had seen me on the street.* They also said she had a sister, a daughter that her dad had raised. She would have to remember that, Emily thought, and find her.

After a few days Emily called her mom. "It's okay here," she said. "The Cree is different from our Cree and I can't really understand when they talk quickly. But it's okay. I'm going to stay and go to school."

She settled into life with her uncle's family in Waswanipi. They lived on Poplar Street in the fourth small grey house.

Emily hadn't been there very long when her grandfather passed away, and her mother visited Waswanipi again for the funeral. Afterwards, Emily and her mother walked out together to the gravesite of Emily's dad. Her mother stood there in front of his gravestone for a long time and cried. Emily stood beside her quietly and put her arm around her. Her mom's tears said what she hadn't been able to say with words: that she had really loved this man whom Emily had never known. His death had hit her very hard. It had taken her breath away.

Over the next years, Emily studied hard and earned her nursing degree. With her dad and grandfather both gone, she had even fewer ties in Waswanipi. She moved to Oujé-Bougoumou and married a guy who lived there. They had one baby, and then another baby, and all the while Emily was studying or working as a nurse and talking on the phone every day with her mom.

Each time Emily was pregnant, she got gestational diabetes, the diabetes that pregnant women sometimes get. She was careful—she remembered her mother and grandfather—but she was a nurse and had studied the disease. She knew that most women with gestational diabetes recover after the baby is born and never get the permanent version that had so affected people she loved. After Emily's first baby, her gestational diabetes went away. After the second baby, it went away too.

But her mom worried. "Be careful, Emily," she said. "It might still get you. Keep a candy in your purse just in case you get weak. And eat properly. And go for a walk. And get some rest!" Emily smiled. Her mom lived with her now, in Oujé-Bougoumou, and even though Emily had kids of her own, her mom still couldn't help but look after her.

In the end, her mom was right: Emily had a third baby, and, after that baby was born, Emily's body did not recover. Her gestational diabetes became exactly the same diabetes—type 2—that her mom and grandfather had.

Gradually, her mom's diabetes worsened and she became very sick. Home dialysis could no longer keep up and she had to leave their home in Oujé-Bougoumou, along with everything she knew, and move to Montréal. There, every three days, she went into the Jewish General Hospital and was hooked up to the much bigger hemodialysis machines that hospitals have. The city—hot and noisy and crowded for anyone—seemed even worse to Emily's mom because she was blind.

Emily had no time to think about her own recent diabetes diagnosis. She packed her things and drove to Montréal to help her mom get used to a new life. Emily's husband, who she could always count on to be supportive, was supportive again. Of course she should be with her mom, he said; he would look after the kids alone.

In the dialysis wing of the hospital, as her mother sat hooked up to the great machines that did the work of kidneys and cleaned her blood, Emily sat with her and watched what was going on around them. A Cree elder in a wheelchair was trying to understand what the doctors and nurses were saying to him but he couldn't speak their languages and they couldn't speak his. He couldn't understand why the nurses were doing the things they were doing, he was afraid of them and of this strange place that smelled of cleaning fluids and sickness, and he couldn't get out of his wheelchair and leave. He said he was waiting for his son to come and help. And he said he was lonely. Surrounded by people, but so lonely.

"You know," her mom said, touching her arm, "In Montréal it's not the diabetes that kills us. It's the sadness. It eats us from inside. We are away from our land and our families when we need them the most. There is no life here. Everywhere you look, it's just more concrete and cars. This is not a place to heal but a place to die." Her face was drawn and heavy with pain.

Everywhere around Emily, Cree people were having a very difficult time. And, although no one spoke of it, Emily knew: they sat in this lonely place of bad memories and bad medicine, immobilized, unable to leave. They were elders, and they had little agency. It was not a good situation.

And then Emily's mother, who had taken many turns for the worse, took a turn for the even-worse. Hemodialysis, even with the big machines, was no longer enough. She needed a new kidney. Her doctor began telephoning around to Emily's family asking each person if they would be tested and, if the blood types matched, would they donate a kidney to Emily's mom. She was still a young woman—only 53. If she had a new kidney, she would live a long time yet.

"Test me," Emily said to the doctor the next time she saw her. "I want to give a kidney to my mother."

The doctor looked at her kindly. "Emily, you're a medical professional. You of all people know that we can't take your kidney even if it is a match. You have diabetes yourself. You need both kidneys."

Emily's mom would have agreed, she knew. She was always urging Emily to take better care of herself. But in that moment Emily would have taken decades off her own life to give her mother more time.

They did not find a match.

Without a new kidney, Emily's mom didn't have much time left. Emily was pregnant just then and needed to go to Chibougamau for a check-up. Her mom was having a good day, so Emily decided to drive to the check-up, and right after it was done, she called her mom from Chibougamau.

"I'm coming back to Montréal now," she said. "The check-up was fine."

Her mom was still feeling well and glad to hear the check-up had gone well.

Very shortly after that, Emily's phone rang again. It was her mother's hospital.

"Hurry down," they said. "Your mom is declining quickly."

"I just spoke to her!" Emily said. But she didn't need to be told twice. She grabbed her stuff and called her husband—she was going to want him there for this.

No sooner had Emily and her husband stepped into her mother's hospital than—of all things—Emily's water broke, and her contractions started.

"Go," her husband said. "I'll stay with your mom."

To deliver her baby, Emily had to go to another hospital. The doctors had said she would need a Caesarean section.

Everything went smoothly, and in a little while Emily had a beautiful baby boy.

She called her husband and told him about their son, and he passed the message on to her mother. Emily's mother smiled as widely as she could and made cradling motions with her arms—she was looking forward to holding her newest grandson and she was very very happy. Emily chatted on the phone with her mom, then, and they talked about the C-section and the new baby. It had been an exciting day, and all was well.

A few minutes later, Emily's husband walked into her hospital room. He had come over from the Jewish hospital where her mom was staying.

In Cree, he said to her, "Your mom has gone home."

Emily's mother had died, a young woman still, in 2009, on the very same day that Emily's son was born.

Emily went back home to Oujé-Bougoumou, at once full of joy about her new son and devastated about her mom. How could she live without her lovely mom? Life had become so complicated. Her son had been born with some medical problems that would correct themselves with time, but he needed extra care now. She looked after him and her other children, she muddled through her routines, she fulfilled her duties at work, and she visited the doctor for check-ups. Emily had diabetes, the doctor reminded her. He gave her pills and told her to look after herself. Emily hardly heard him. She didn't have time to look after herself. And her mom, her lovely mom, was gone. What was the *point*?

Once, while Emily was doing a nursing placement in the hospital, a virus attacked her joints. For a while, any kind of movement was painful. She went home, still sick with the virus, and took time off work to recover. One afternoon, she tried to get up from the couch to go to the bedroom. She couldn't get to her feet. She was too weak.

"Here Mom, let us help you."

Two of her sons, still young children, were there, right away, one on each side of her. They helped Emily to her feet. From there she could make her way to the bedroom, leaning heavily on counters and walls.

Just before she closed the door behind her, she caught the expressions on their faces. They were terrified. Their mother was so sick. What if she didn't get better? What if something happened to her? What then?

They need me!, she thought. *They feel about me the way I felt about my mom!*

It was a new thought. This virus—she knew it would run its course and she would recover. But she also had diabetes. And, unless she changed a few things, it would eventually make her as sick as it had made her mom and grandfather. From that she would not be able to recover.

I have to make myself healthier for them.

Gradually, over that summer, Emily recovered from the virus and began to feel better. One day, she knew that the time had come to do what her mom had always asked of her, to take better care of her health.

She would start by making a plan. She hobbled to the shelf with her nursing books, pulled down a few, opened the drawer for paper and a pen, then made a list of things she could do to be healthier.

It was a long list: Keep a positive attitude. Take meds. Limit sugar and salt. Check blood sugar. Eat carefully. Exercise every day, even when there's no time for exercise. Keep a positive attitude. And never let up.

Emily, now healthy and living with diabetes, has never forgotten the elders she met in the dialysis wing of the Jewish hospital in Montréal. They knew, as Cree have known for many generations, that they heal better on their own land and amongst their own people. Emily works in public health, as part of a group figuring out how to bring wellness into the communities of Eeyou Istchee for people of all ages.

She still misses her mom. She lies awake at night, sometimes, thinking about her. Like diabetes, that longing will never go away.

12

The Story of Leonard House of Chisasibi

ONE day, when Leonard was small, he and his mother left their teepee, heading to the right towards the rising sun, to check the snares. His mother was a marvel with small game. She knew just where the animals came and how they behaved. In one area, at the bottom of a hill, she showed Leonard how to set a snare to catch a rabbit. Further on, in a cluster of trees, she showed him how to tie it another way, with a loop at the end of a long pole, to catch a grouse around the neck. And if they came to a snare holding game that was still alive, she showed him how to kill it, quickly and mercifully. She dropped the fresh catch in the pack on Leonard's back or in the bag on her own shoulder and they walked on to the next snare. They walked and walked. At the end of the day, both packs heavy with game, they came again upon their teepee—and it was on their right side. They had gone in a big circle, but Leonard thought she had taken him around the world. His parents had descended from chiefs, he knew; no wonder she could do such things. He lay down for a nap and watched through falling eyelids as his mother skinned and prepared the meat into the most wonderful dishes. Such food, such wealth, such comfort.

For the rest of his life, Leonard would love small game best of all.

At lunchtime in the Fort George Anglican Residential School, back when a whole town lived out on the island, the kids lined up as they always did. There was a line for washing hands and another line for getting food scooped into their bowls. Full of energy after sitting all morning, the kids bounced and the teachers were frazzled and distracted trying to keep order. Leonard approached a supervisor.

"Please sir, may I go to the outhouse?"

"Yes Leonard. Put on your coat, it's cold outside. And come right back." The teacher hardly glanced his way.

Leonard put on his coat and boots, his scarf and his mittens, and headed out the door towards the row of outhouses. He even went into a toilet. Then he opened the door a crack to see if the coast was clear, and he ran into the trees behind the outhouses, away from school property. He ran towards the town, keeping to the treed areas, where adults wouldn't see him and send him back to school. He wove this way and that, and, in a little while, he was at his own house.

The door was padlocked. No one was home. Leonard snuck around his house to the east side where there was a large window made up of many smaller sections. He picked up a rock and used it to smash a hole in the smallest part of the window. With his mitts he cleared away the rest of the glass, and then he wiggled through into his house.

The house was stone cold. His father was out on the land, getting food for the family, and, when he was gone, his mother had trouble getting wood for the house. She spent her waking hours working for the school board or hunting for food and had no time to chop down a tree, nor extra money to buy chopped wood from a neighbour. There could be no fire to warm the house until his father returned. Still, Leonard was happier here, in his stone-cold house, than in school where those teachers could do anything. Sure, they would feed him and bandage a cut if he hurt himself, but they could also slap him around for no reason at all. Or worse—the

Anglican principal there invited the young boys, one at a time, to go "hunting" off school property, but the boys soon learned that he had something else on his mind altogether. You never knew what was coming at school. Leonard kept his coat on, wrapped up in a blanket, and slept.

Late in the evening, after dark, his mother came home and found him there. She shook him awake.

"Leonard! What are you doing here? You'll catch cold!"

"I want to be here," he said.

"Oh Leonard." She hugged him to herself. She still smelled like the outside. "You have to go back. You'll get sick if you're not warm. I can't keep you warm."

He begged her to stay in his safe home, in her warm company. Being cold, or having a cold, those things didn't bother him. But she took him back to school anyways.

It was always like that. He ran home from Fort George Anglican Residential School many times, and every time his mother took him back because she could not afford to keep him warm and she had already lost so many children to illness. And later, at other schools in Rouyn-Noranda and in Moose Factory and in La Tuque, Leonard cried and cried, wanting to be home with his safe parents where there was love. He learned then how to cut them out of his head, how to not think about them and their ways. Just so that they would be out of his mind. So that the wounds would be less raw. He thought instead about his fine hockey team, and how he loved to play. Or about the girl he liked and how he had fainted when he asked her out. (On his way to the floor, he heard her say no. When he came to, she was kneeling over him. "I'm so sorry!" she said. "I didn't think my answer would make you collapse." "It wasn't you," he said. "It was the effort.")

Being taken away and put in a place where the people in charge could do anything to him—it was terrifying. And who could he tell about the things that went on there? They never talked about residential school in his house. He couldn't tell anyone from the government because they were behind it. He couldn't tell anyone from the church or the school because they were behind it too. He could exist there only if they permitted it. They could make any laws they wanted.

Many years later, Leonard would have a man paint a picture of his house on Fort George Island, his house where he had been safe and didn't cry with fear and longing, where his parents had loved him.

Leonard was the youngest kid of many. Ten or twelve, maybe more, he was never sure. Through his whole life, it was just him and his parents. The other kids were all gone, taken away to residential school or when they got sick with tuberculosis, and they never came back. Once, when Leonard was grown, an old man recognized him and said "Your brother is on the island at the mouth of Roggan River. He died there and they buried him in the ground." That was all the man said. Leonard didn't know how old his brother had been, nor even his name. Only that his parents had buried a child, his brother, at the mouth of Roggan River and had never ever talked about it.

His mother, genius of snaring small game and of walking around the world in a day, worked for the school board until she died in '72. Leonard never knew of what she died, but it probably had something to do with all the things she had to go through. And being cold, so cold, for so many years.

Big changes came to the Eeyou Istchee and to Fort George. In the 1970s, the Province of Québec began the James Bay Hydroelectric Project, one of the world's biggest hydroelectric generating systems, on Cree land. In the courtrooms, the Grand Council of the Crees duked it out with the provincial government over land rights, and, when the dust had settled, the dam building began. Leonard had a family by then and he found work on the dams to support them.

He went out as a labourer, driving dump trucks or shovelling stone, doing whatever needed to be done, but he wanted to be a large-machine operator.

One day, the superintendent approached him.

"Hey Leonard, you wanna drive a big tractor?"

"Big tractor!?"

"Yep. You'll be a large-machine operator."

"Yes!" The big machines were mostly operated by white guys. Leonard would be one of the first Cree large-machine operators on the project.

The superintendent led him over to where the big machines sat when they weren't being used. They walked past machine after machine to the very end of the row. There sat a small tractor, the smallest kind of tractor they had on the project, not much bigger than a lawnmower.

"Here's your big tractor, Leonard."

Everybody laughed then, including Leonard. That was how he became an operator. After a long time of working on that small tractor, Leonard moved up to the big tractors and did finally become a large-machine operator—but he hated it. He hated it so much that he asked to move back to his little tractor. (And he laughed at that too.)

For years Leonard worked on the dams, building up reservoirs and cofferdams that quickly swallowed the slow-worn beauty of the La Grande river valleys. He loved the precision of the work, the way each dam would be built in layers, with carefully levelled sand and stone and a peak at the centre. He worked through springs and summers and autumns. In winters, he went out into the bush, lived off the land with his father, and learned what he could about traditional life.

Once the dams were built, the government began to relocate the whole town of Fort George 14 kilometres inland to Chisasibi. As soon as the dam project would begin producing power, the island on which Fort George stood would begin to erode, they thought, and eventually split in two as the water wore a chasm down the centre. It wouldn't be safe to live there anymore. It was a shame, really. There was an area on one side of the island where the river had always slowed and, in the summers of his childhood, Leonard and his friends had gone swimming there. They weren't supposed to but of course they did anyways. The dams had their own beauty, sure, and they brought money to the Cree, but now all this would disappear, swallowed by the diverted La Grande. How would his kids, for whom he was doing all this work, ever understand him if they could never swim there nor see his old house, the place where he had felt most loved?

But there could be no time for nostalgia. Moving the town was employment. Leonard had to cut these thoughts out of his head. Again he worked for the government, this time as a house inspector. After each house was uprooted from the island, it was set on a flatbed, the flatbed driven onto a barge, and the barge taken across the river. Then the house and flatbed were driven off the barge to the new location in Chisasibi. There, on its new foundation, each house had to be inspected for safety and any necessary repairs made before the families could move in. Leonard walked into 211 resettled houses, poking into corners, checking the windows, testing the wiring, peering into crawlspaces and attics. His own house was gone. Now it was his job to make sure the other houses were safe and would keep people warm in the subarctic winter.

When the relocation business came to an end, Leonard bought a building, hired a good mechanic, and began running a garage. To pay for the building and mechanic, he worked for a government economic development agency.

All these years he was busy working to provide for his family. Busy thinking how strange it was that he, who had lost so much to the white government, had worked so much for same government. Busy starting to drink, and then busy drinking some more. Busy being frustrated with his own people, who should have come together during the time of relocation to make decisions as a community and who instead imposed rules and structures and methods that made Leonard think again of residential school ways. And busy drinking some more. Busy thinking about his marriage that was sometimes difficult and drinking some more. Busy thinking about his mom and dad and drinking some more. In that whole time, Leonard never thought once that his pancreas might be giving up, that he would get diabetes.

It was 1985 and Leonard was so tired he could hardly get through a day. All he wanted was sleep. And every day that week he had stopped by the Northern, picked up a jug of apple juice or orange, and slugged the whole thing back like it was nothing. And still he was thirsty. His wife would bring him a pitcher of water and he'd drink the whole thing. He'd go to the washroom then, pee it all out, come back to the kitchen and beg for more water—and go back to bed.

"Leonard," she said, after a few days of this. "You have to go to the clinic. I saw something on TV. If you're thirsty and sleepy like this, you have to go to the clinic."

At the clinic, Leonard heard for the first time that his blood sugar level was extremely high and he had diabetes. They gave him bottles of the insulin medication and some long needles and taught him how to fill the syringe from the bottle and sink it into fat on his stomach or thigh. And they told him he'd be injecting himself every day for the rest of his life. They gave him a long list of things he was supposed to change in his life: more exercise, more game, less stress, less dumplings and bannock, less bread and salt, less sugar and juice, and, because alcohol was sugar, less alcohol. Way less alcohol.

Now, he was angry. Who were these people to impose these rules? He enjoyed his drink. Who were they to tell him to stop? Who were they to try and make him change so many things? What more would he have to go through in this life? If only he could escape to an outhouse and then run home.

For a long time, Leonard was angry. He didn't make any of the big changes the doctors told him to make. He took his medicine when his wife brought it to him and ate what she put in front of him but he didn't put his own effort into doing what the doctor said he should do.

At home, his wife overhauled the family diet. She emptied the house of sugars and sweets—even at Christmas there would be no sweets—she began to cook without salt, and she made sure the freezer was filled with the small game that Leonard so loved and that was healthy for people with diabetes. Every day, she brought him his insulin and watched him take it. When Leonard was feeling down from his diabetes, she reminded him of good things in his life, things he could still do. She worked to make the house a place of calm so that stress would not drive up Leonard's sugar levels and make him sick. When his levels dropped so low that he slipped into a coma, she tried to get sugar into his mouth to bring the levels back up and revive him. And when that didn't work, she called the ambulance and waited. When the ambulance showed up with the wrong stretcher, she waited, nerves wracking, while they went back to get a different one. Months later, when he went into a second coma, she called the ambulance again, and waited, nerves wracking again, and they showed up with the wrong stretcher again. (On the third coma, they got it right.) She taught her kids and grandkids what to do if he slipped into a coma. All the while Leonard continued to drink. His blood sugar levels would spike and then drop very low—and up and down and up and down and up and down.

For years, things went on like this. Being sick so often was taking much away from his life and the day came that Leonard had finally had enough. His drinking was causing so many problems. It was getting in the way of life.

Leonard got his alcohol addiction under control by getting hooked on something else: around 1990, he took on the habit of reading the Christian bible. Before he had reached for alcohol every time he felt bad, and he felt bad a lot, so he had often reached for alcohol. Now, under this new addiction, when he thought about his mom so cold in her house, or his times at the Fort George Anglican Residential School, or the difficult times in his marriage, or his disappointment in people, or the ways in which the government had complicated his life—all the things that had once made him drink—now they were not his problem. The more he read his bible, the more he began to enjoy it, to crave it, and the less he needed to drink (he stopped drinking altogether around '95) and the less he worried about his illness. Diabetes existed, and he was reminded of that every day when he injected himself with insulin, but he no longer worried about it. He had been in three comas, he knew his diabetes was serious, but he no longer worried about it. The ways of his people had changed so much since his time on the land as a child. His kids would have money but never the wealth of his rich young life. They would never see his old swimming hole nor walk around the world in an afternoon. But he no longer worried about it.

It wasn't an easy change to make. There was so much to forgive. And it got *lonely.* Leonard had no church community— church rules and structures and repetitions were not for him. He wished the people around him understood how he felt fulfilled and loved again every time he opened his bible and wished they would feel the same. But they called him a Cree word that means "the person with the strange religion," and said his ways were not for them. They took no interest in what he had to say. Sometimes

Leonard longed for the bush, for its peace and solitude that was never lonely, but he couldn't go: his insulin had to be kept at a specific temperature to be effective and there were no refrigerators out in the bush. In these times of frustration, he reached for his bible. God had his own laws and could do anything he wanted. When Leonard's time came to die, he would die. Until then, he would live as well as he could and not worry about it.

Leonard's wife still works hard at home to keep the freezer full of small game and to manage his medication and traditional diet so that Leonard doesn't get sick. And Leonard works on his faith.

13

The Story of Elizabeth Bell Tayler* of Wemindji

ELIZABETH Bell Tayler is a receptionist. Every morning she goes to work and opens the office and makes a big pot of coffee. All the other workers come by her desk for a cup, to see if there were any messages left for them overnight, or just to say hi. They're all so nice. Interesting people. She spends the morning taking phone calls and taking care of office matters.

Then the afternoons come. They are unbearably slow. Elizabeth gets restless. Years ago, she walked all the time out by the dam, along the Maquatua River, and by Paint Hills Bay. It's beautiful there. Even in summer, when blackflies are everywhere, she would ignore the bugs and go for a walk. Now, in her office in the long afternoons, her bum wants so badly to move. She wants so badly to do something. The river calls to her. But she's the receptionist and she's supposed to sit there and wait for the phone to ring.

And so she does. She reaches for *The Nation* or something else to read. With every hour of sitting, she can feel her blood pressure rise.

Names and details in this story have been changed to protect identities.

After work Elizabeth goes home and makes supper. It'd sure be nice to walk out by the river then, but usually there's someone who needs looking after. Women are supposed to put family first. Her husband is a good one. He takes care of his own diabetes medication so she doesn't have to worry about that, and he's good company. He even helps out around the house. He does his part. But still, he needs feeding and his clothes need washing, and, well, Elizabeth takes better care of him than she does of herself.

And Elizabeth raised her four daughters. They needed all the love and attention that kids usually need. They went through elementary school and all graduated from high school and got themselves jobs. Good kids.

After they were mostly grown and Elizabeth had less childcare, her mom needed more help with her diabetes. Elizabeth looked after her and administered injections. She was the one to poke the needle into the insulin bottle, pull back on the plunger, measure out the proper amount of insulin, and poke it into her mother's stomach or thigh. It was kind of fun. She would probably be a good nurse, she realized, but she wouldn't be good at having diabetes. When Elizabeth watched her sister inject herself with insulin, she thought *I don't ever want to be poking myself every time I eat and I could never keep track of all those rules.* But she'd be a good nurse.

Elizabeth's mom died in 2011, and that was about the time that one of her adult daughters started going through a tough time: she had diabetes too, so her blood sugar could get very high and she would get so sick, but she didn't want to admit it or believe what the doctor said. Other things were going on in her daughter's life then too, on top of the diabetes—marriage problems, addictions. Elizabeth was always trying to help out. She would look after the grandkids so that her daughter could have a break and take care of herself. It's the sort of thing grandmothers are supposed to do.

After that, the childcare never really stopped. Elizabeth looks after one or another of her grandkids almost every evening. You're not supposed to say no to your own daughter just because you want to go for a walk out along the river. Elizabeth knows her daughter has work to do too. And she loves those kids. She loves spending time with them, but it's sure not what she expected. Her grandkids have gaming consoles and smartphones and all that stuff. So much brain clutter.

"You know," she says to them, "when I was young, my parents would put us in a boat and take us out to an island in James Bay. Dad would build a smoking rack from saplings and twine. Then he'd go fishing and me and my mom would clean all the fish he caught and drape them over the rack. Underneath we'd build a wet smoky fire and that smoke would rise up and soak into the fish and preserve them so that we could eat them in winter. And we would go swimming at that island and canoeing and do all kinds of things. We had so much fun. We didn't need any gaming consoles or smartphones. We didn't want to be inside huddled away from the sun. It was so peaceful, that life."

Her grandkids look at her kindly, like they might feel sorry for her, and they say, "Sure Grandma. That's nice." And go back to their gaming. It's not what she expected at all, but it's nice all the same.

Elizabeth spends so much time with the grandkids that she notices things. Like her granddaughter, a nice girl, trying to tell her mom about another girl in school who had been cruel to her. Her mom, Elizabeth's daughter, didn't seem to pay attention. And then later, when they were all in town, her granddaughter pointed out the bully and said "Look Mom, that's the girl who hurt me," and still her mom didn't do anything. So Elizabeth comforted her grand-daughter later, and told her that she had noticed and paid attention and thought that bullying was just awful. Now the girl doesn't tell those things to her own mother, she tells Elizabeth.

The other night, her grandkids were sleeping in their room at Elizabeth's house. In the night, through a crack in the door, Elizabeth saw her granddaughter get up to use the washroom and walk back to her room. But then she turned around and went to Grandma Elizabeth's bed and stood there, beside Elizabeth's bed, in the dark.

"What's wrong?" Elizabeth asked.

"I can't sleep," she said.

"Are you worried about school?"

"No."

"What is it then?"

"I'm afraid of dying. Does it hurt to die?"

Elizabeth couldn't believe what she was hearing. Since when did seven-year-olds worry about death?

"Don't think about that when you go to bed," Elizabeth said. "Are you scared to sleep alone?"

"Yeah."

"Do you want to sleep with me and Grandpa?"

"Okay."

Elizabeth moved over to make room for her granddaughter in the bed, and they snuggled together under the blankets and prayed and the girl fell asleep.

But Elizabeth stayed awake. What did it mean that a seven-year-old lay awake at night thinking of death? To whom could Elizabeth talk about this? Was the girl worried because Elizabeth had taken her to the funeral of her own mother when she had died of diabetes and the girl had seen the corpse there in the coffin? Or was this just part of childhood now, something kids were supposed to do, like gaming consoles and smartphones?

Then Elizabeth thought back to another time she was awake in the night, years and years ago. One of the first times she had gone along to the bush with her parents. Her dad had packed his sleeping bag and food and had canoed to another camp with his brother to catch beaver. Elizabeth and her sister had stayed behind with their mother and it was their job to make sure the fire kept burning all night. That night their mother woke up because she was sweating so much under the covers—she was soaked, her clothes were soaked, even her feather blanket was soaked—and it wasn't warm outside at all. Elizabeth and her sister helped her change her clothes under the blanket and they were as wet as clothes on laundry day. Was her mother already diabetic then? Elizabeth lay awake wondering. Were those night sweats early symptoms, way out there in the bush?

And what of her own diabetes? Almost ten years ago, Elizabeth went to the clinic for a check-up and everything was fine. The next day, she got a phone call from the clinic pharmacy.

"You forgot to pick up your pills," the lady said.

"What pills? The nurse said I was fine and could go home."

"Your diabetes pills."

"Oh that's a mix-up," Elizabeth said. "Two of my daughters have diabetes, and my mother and husband have diabetes and a couple of my sisters do too—the pills are for one of them."

"No," the clinic lady said, "I have your chart here. The pills are definitely for you."

And that's how Elizabeth learned she had diabetes.

One time, long before that, Elizabeth was walking out by the dam and looking back at her lovely village. She had felt so weak she could hardly stand—she had needed something, some kind of fuel, to keep going. She forced herself along, one step at a time, and made it home. After that she always carried a sliced apple when she went out walking. Had that been low blood sugar? The beginning of something wrong? An early diabetes symptom, like her mom's night sweats?

Beside her in bed, Elizabeth's granddaughter snored a little. On the other side of the girl lay Elizabeth's husband. Sometimes he got fed up with raising kids again, impatient with the ways they always make noise, always need *something*. He and Elizabeth had already done this once and they had looked after their own kids when they had them. (Or, at least, Elizabeth had.) He said to Elizabeth that their daughter should take responsibility for the choices she made, for the children she birthed. Elizabeth agreed with him then—sometimes it would be nice to spend a day shopping. Or go for a walk out by the river. But those kids need looking after. If she didn't do it, who would? So Elizabeth got into the habit of sending her tired husband to work, or to visit a friend, and she would take care of the kids. And after he had had a short break, he remembered how much he loved them and he could be patient again. Sometimes it's so much work to please everyone.

Then Elizabeth thought about boats. It'd be nice to go for a boat ride. You can just sit still on the water and fish, and later eat the fish you caught. So much tastier than food from cardboard boxes. When she was a kid, they went fishing often, but now, they almost never go. And then Elizabeth thought again about walking out by the river, and finally, finally, she fell asleep.

All her life, Elizabeth has heard that a woman is supposed to look after the people in her family, to put their needs first, and she has done that. A while ago, the doctor told her that, for some people, diabetes can be brought on by the stress of everyday living. She believes it, she can feel it in her own body. He even implied that Elizabeth should take better care of herself. Another thing to feel guilty about.

But really, what more can she do? When so many people need something from her, when she doesn't have the time to plan meals carefully nor to police every morsel that goes into her mouth, when she doesn't have the time to memorize every one of the dozens of complicated diabetes rules, when she lies awake at night worrying about the people she loves, when she doesn't have time even to go for a walk out by the river, when there just isn't enough time in the day—really, what more can she do?

Stories We Heard Along the Way: Elders

An elderly Cree woman was sitting outside in Chibougamau when a young man ran by and grabbed her purse and tried to run away with it. She held on. He tugged harder. She held on. He tugged harder still. She held on. Finally he gave up and ran away. Later, she said, "If he'd known how many moose hides my hands have stretched over the years, he wouldn't even have tried."

•

A Cree grandma walked back to her car after an evening event but stopped because several wolves were circling it. She yelled at them in Cree to get away from her car. They turned around and looked at her, but didn't move. She yelled at them in English. They didn't move. She threw stuff at them. Still, they didn't move. Then she picked up a lodgepole pine that lay by the road and waved it back and forth. The wolves realized that a Cree grandma who could wield a whole tree should not be messed with. They ran away.

•

An older Cree man was in the hospital in Val-d'Or for a while. Nothing in his body worked quite as well as it once had and he was beginning to go blind. Eventually, the hospital discharged him and his family came to drive him home. On the drive home, the sun was already below the horizon when five geese flew overhead, honking loudly. "Stop the truck," the old man said, "and hand me that gun." The truck pulled over, and, out of the back of the pickup, the old man raised the gun. Bam! Bam! Bam! Bam! Bam! Five shots and five geese fell out of the sky, just like that. He must have been really tired of hospital food—not even failing vision nor the darkness of evening could stop him from getting a traditional goose dinner.

•

The town of Wemindji was looking to build an airport. Some experts came up from the South and did topographical surveys looking for the perfect site. There were all kinds of requirements: it had to have a flat area about 5000 feet long and 300 feet wide for the runway, it had to be on stable soil, and so forth. After they had spent hundreds of thousands of dollars on six months of studies, the experts from the South announced that they had finally found the perfect site— but it was 30 kilometres out of town. A council meeting was held in English to discuss building an airport so far away. One of the elders there didn't speak English. "What are they talking about?" he asked his friend sitting beside him. His friend translated and explained that the only land they could find for an airport was 30 kilometres away. "What kind of land do they need?" he asked. His friend explained all the requirements. The old man listened carefully, and said, "I know a place like that just one kilometre outside of town." The place the elder suggested is the site of Wemindji's airport today.

14

The Story of Jennifer Gloria Lowpez* of Waswanipi

IN 2007 or so, things at Jennifer Gloria Lowpez's home were not going so great. One night she slugged back some pills, lots of pills, and went out to a bar where she drank some beer and then some wine and then some rum and then some vodka. Then she grabbed an empty beer bottle, broke it against the bar, and cut herself right across a vein. She crumpled in a heap and her spirit lifted and left her body that was still bleeding out on the grimy pub floor.

Someone was saying into her ear, "Stay Jennifer, your kids need you." But kids or no kids, it was time to go. Finally, it was time to go.

Jennifer woke up in the Chibougamau hospital. Someone, probably that person who spoke in her ear, had called an ambulance. Her boyfriend, who had told her that no one could ever love someone as fat and ugly as Jennifer, sat in the chair by the bed. She turned over on her side and faced away from him.

If only the suicide had worked.

In January 2010, the doctor told Jennifer she had diabetes.

*Names and details in this story have been changed to protect identities.

She cried and cried and cried. What was diabetes anyways? Didn't people with diabetes go blind and get infections and then amputation after amputation until they didn't have any arms or legs left? Jennifer's heels were always cracked: if anyone's foot was gonna get infected and have to be sawed off, it'd be hers. And then it'd be her other foot and then one arm and then the other and soon she wouldn't have any limbs and would die a horrible pus-filled death.

The nutritionist who talked to Jennifer about diabetes kept handing her Kleenex for her tears but didn't really explain much. Still, Jennifer started taking diabetes pills because she was supposed to. They made her lose a few pounds, but not many. She still felt like a Christmas tree. A terrified Christmas tree.

The good thing was that comfort was available every single day. Three meals plus two chocolate bars a day, plus snacks of cookies and poutine between meals, plus a big Costco bag of chips and dip along with a couple of bottles of Pepsi with her kids every night, plus a six-pack of beer and a glass or two of wine gradually emptied over dinner and through the evening after the kids had gone to bed. And then, every ten days or so, Jennifer would binge-drink to get good and wasted for two solid days. The bingeing bugged her kids, but Jennifer needed comfort, escape. Oh, and cocaine. Cocaine definitely made her feel better. It made her feel better about seven or eight times a week.

A few months after her diabetes diagnosis, in spring of 2011, Jennifer went with her family to Marineland and stood in line with them to go on a ride. Her boyfriend was standing in front of her, joking with the kids in line, and Jennifer was looking him over and thinking. He was gone at work half the time and he was hot. Even after eighteen years of being together on and off, he was hot. It was his blue eyes that did it.

But something weird was going on. These days he was acting even more moody and strange and secretive than usual: he had accused Jennifer of cheating on him which was the most ridiculous thing in the world because, as he sometimes pointed out, no one would ever want her—so, you know, how could she cheat? And their daughter was acting strange and secretive too. Everything was awkward and uncomfortable all around. Something was up.

Their turn at the ride came and Jennifer stepped into the enclosure to sit in her seat—but the ride gate couldn't latch behind her. It just banged into her Christmas tree ass which was, for everyone there to see, obviously too fat for the ride.

"I'm sorry ma'am," the ride operator said gently. "The safety regulations won't allow us to take you on this ride. But if you walk up there," and he pointed to where the ride ended, "you can meet your family when they step off."

He was polite and spoke softly.

Jennifer nodded, stepped down from the enclosure, and headed up to where she would meet her family. She wanted to disappear.

Sure, she had a hard time moving her body—just looking at a hill and thinking about walking up would make her cry. Sure, she was a big girl—she joked about her Christmas tree ass louder than anyone in the room. A big ass is what happens when you start having kids at 18 and keep on having them until there are four of 'em, and then you get a job at a grocery store to help pay the bills and you're surrounded by junk food all the time, and you eat it because you're so friggin' exhausted from chasing after your kids and you need energy to keep chasing after them. Okay okay, she was 300 lbs and that was really big. But too big for an amusement park ride? She really wished her kids hadn't seen that.

When they got home from their Marineland vacation from hell, she found out her handsome boyfriend and father of her four kids was leaving her. And then she found out that he—who had accused her of cheating—had been seeing another woman for a year already. That through the whole family vacation at Marineland he had been telling his girlfriend he had already left Jennifer and the kids. And that he, who had always said he didn't want more kids, had gotten that other girl pregnant. And, worst of all, that he had made their daughter lie to Jennifer to help cover up his affair.

Her handsome blue-eyed boyfriend was kind of an asshole.

It was a lot to take in.

It was *a lot* to take in and it kind of got under Jennifer's skin.

She reached for some chocolate-bar comfort—and stopped. Food wasn't really what she wanted. She went to her cupboard and reached instead for the vodka bottle, but she didn't really want that either. Maybe some blow? That always made her feel amazing. She picked up the phone to call her dealer and set it back down on the cradle. Cocaine wasn't it either.

What she wanted, what she really really wanted, was to go for a walk. And that was as big a surprise as her boyfriend cheating on her.

Jennifer tied on her most comfortable shoes and walked to the track and began to go around. She was a big girl and she couldn't walk effortlessly like her kids did. She had to shift her weight to the one side, swing her leg around to take a step, and then shift it to the other side for the next step. By the end of the first lap, she was sweating. By the end of the fifth lap, she was exhausted. By the end of the tenth, she was half dead. Still, she kept walking until she had gone around that friggin' track twenty friggin' times.

And the next day, she did it again.

You know what, she thought to herself as she walked, *this walking thing sucks. I'm gonna do more of it. Twenty laps a day, every day, for one month. And then I'll quit.*

While she walked, she thought about her boyfriend. Sure, he was Mr. Blue Eyes and a whole lot of women wanted him, but handsome isn't everything. Now that he was gone, his blue eyes were gone too, but she sure didn't miss hearing all that fat-and-ugly shit he hurled at her every now and then. The sound waves in her house were a whole lot happier without all that. She actually didn't miss him at all. Money was gonna be a problem now—she and her kids would have to go on welfare until she found other ways to make ends meet. That was stressful. Thinking about it made her cry. Remembering all the ways he had been mean to her made her cry.

The good thing was that even with the crying, walking was getting easier and sucking less. So she started walking to work every day too, and anywhere she needed to go that was in walking distance, always avoiding shortcuts—if a path cut across a yard, she walked around to collect twenty extra steps.

By the end of the month, she thought she might like to keep walking. It gave her time to think. Cleared her head. Felt okay.

Walking made Jennifer hungry, so, naturally, she started thinking about junk food.

Okay, when she really thought about it, she had to admit she ate more of it than most people. Maybe she could cut back, a little less of it every day.

Or she could try one month without it—

Ohhh man.

That was not gonna be easy. One month of walking and sweating seemed a whole lot easier than one month without chocolate bars and cookies and chips and pop.

But she was gonna have to try.

The first month of walking had been a challenge. The first month of no junk food was friggin' brutal. She started inventing tricks to get through the month. She froze water and crushed the ice into a slurpee so that she could still go through the motions of drinking pop, even if there was no pop there. But, without all the sugar she was used to, she got the shakes every afternoon. She would shake so badly that she couldn't still her hands enough to hold a pen or type. She had to ease up on herself then and have a Pepsi. Immediately the shakes would subside.

This was full-on addiction withdrawal. This was what heroin junkies went through when they went off smack. Worse, because heroin detox lasted a few days, a week at most and, after three weeks then four weeks, Jennifer's detox symptoms were still coming on strong. When the first month was up, she still really wanted junk food, so she had some. Then she figured she had come this far, might as well keep goin'. Once a month she would have a junk food night with her kids so that she wouldn't feel deprived, but the other nights she might as well keep on eating healthy. What did she have to lose? Jennifer's detox symptoms, though, lasted beyond that first month and the next and the next. They lasted for *six friggin' months*.

She thought about that as she walked. Did other folks around here know that sugar was a nasty ol' addiction? Had she missed that class in school? Was she the only one who had always thought junk food was, you know, *food*? Was she the only one who had never known?

One morning, a while after she had quit junk food, Jennifer woke with a bad-ass hangover. Headache, puking, dry mouth, the works.

She hung over the toilet, heaving out the dregs of her unhappy gut, and thinking.

She sure had had plenty of hangovers in her day. She had been drinking at the same level, the teenager-trying-to-get-good-and-wasted level, for twenty years, since she had been 18 years old. Two or three times a month for twenty years plus a few extra-intense years along the way—

Over *a thousand* hangovers.

She was sick of hangovers. And of how her drinking upset her kids. When she went out drinking, she would leave the younger kids in the care of the eldest, who was old enough to babysit, but the younger ones resented having the oldest be the boss of them, and the oldest hated being in that difficult position with younger kids who wouldn't listen. It was hard for everybody, all around.

That's it, Jennifer thought, looking into the toilet bowl. *No more.*

Now she knew what to do. She could do one month without booze. Well, maybe not totally without—this wasn't AA. She would savor a glass of something every week or so, sip it slowly, but for a month there would be no more getting wasted, and no more six-pack of beer every evening.

Besides, she didn't need it so much. Now that she didn't have to listen to her ex hurling insults at her, now that her body didn't feel sick all the time, she didn't need escape. Her life was beginning to feel like something worth living, something worth sticking around for.

Cutting out most drinking wasn't exactly easy—she had heavy liquor cravings for a month, and light cravings for a few months after that—but it was manageable. And wouldn't you know, at the end of a month without a single hangover, she liked how she felt and didn't want to get wasted again.

She wasn't *quitting*—she didn't like that word because *quitting* sounded like she might begin again, like the folks who quit smoking for a couple of weeks and then took it up again. She was *stopping*. Full *stop*. Done. No more.

Not another binge or hangover in her entire life.

Soon after the end of booze, Jennifer went to the clinic for her diabetes follow-up. The nutritionist went on and on again. There were some Science words and then Jennifer was supposed to do this and not supposed to do that and she was doing this wrong and that wrong and she should eat more of this and less of that and blah blah blah blah blah blah blah.

She walked home from the clinic and thought about it.

Really, it was just all negativity and confusion and it wasn't helping at all. She didn't want someone else telling her what she was doing wrong or what to eat or that she was too fat—she'd had enough of all that with ol' Blue Eyes.

That's it, she thought, *No more nutritionist, no more diabetes appointments*. She would keep on doing stuff that made her feel better and would keep on not doing stuff that made her feel worse. She'd check in with the doctor every now and again, like she always had, for general check-ups. But not for diabetes appointments.

Quitting the clinic was easy. She wasn't gonna need a month to wean herself off of that. She could do it in one day.

There was just one more habit to get under control. Beautiful, beautiful blow. Jennifer was still using every day and she wasn't entirely sure she wanted to quit. Not because she feared withdrawal— she didn't—but because cocaine felt amazing. Even after all these years it felt amazing. When she had started walking and had stopped junk food and then drinking, she had always eventually felt better for it. But she was pretty sure that she felt a whole lot better high on blow than she ever would feel if she were clean.

Still, she could try it for a month. She'd probably sleep better. It'd be good for the kids, too, to see her try. To see her not be good at something and then try to get better at it.

And maybe she could still do a line every few weeks or so.

The first couple of days brought some intense cravings. Not as bad as the sugar cravings had been when she cut out junk food, but still, pretty bad. Jennifer went through the motions. She went to work and looked after her kids and hung out with her friends, but, through it all, she thought about sniffing back lines of white powder and that electric buzz when it hit your brain, when you knew that for a few minutes everything would be all right. And for the first week or so, she was so cranky that any little thing would set her off.

Sometimes, in the evenings, she smoked a bit of weed to take the edge off. It did the trick and didn't make her heart race nor her eyes look weird.

After a few weeks, she snorted a line of blow. Surprisingly, the high wasn't really all that great. She still craved it, of course—it was cocaine—but she didn't really need it. It wasn't worth what it took out of her. She was done with it. Without rehab or treatment or AA or even talking with an elder about it, she had brought her cocaine addiction under control.

And stopping blow had been easier than stopping junk food. That was something to think about too.

Jennifer found work eventually. Financially things levelled out at home. She kept walking and thinking.

Half the time, she was thinking about the toilet. She felt so much better now, but her body was still getting used to all the changes she had made and it had become anemic—she had had to go on iron pills and they plugged her up like a drain full of hair. So, at work, when everybody else was thinking about a drink and a barbeque after work, Jennifer was thinking about the toilet. And when she walked around the track, she thought about it more: *When I go to the toilet, is it actually gonna come?* The doctor said that would fix itself eventually. And it did.

The other half the time, she was thinking about other things. Her cousin, who had been one of her favourite people, had committed suicide and there were a few things about that whole situation that just didn't make sense.

She thought about her kids too. "Mom, you're killin' me!" her son would say when dinner would again be something healthy with lots of vegetables, but he would eat it anyways. She was a better mom now that she was healthier. She liked her kids more and had more patience with the ways they were kids.

Sometimes she still thought about her ex-boyfriend. He was gone, moved to another community to be with his new family.

Jennifer was much smaller than she had once been. People kept asking her if she was starving herself. (She wasn't.) Even her doctor had had to pick up his jaw from the floor when she walked into his office. But she hadn't lost the weight for ol' Blue Eyes. She had done the work for herself to feel good in her own body. She would never have been able to do it if he had been around.

On one of those walks, half thinking about the toilet and half thinking about her new life, she realized that she wouldn't take Blue Eyes back. She had seen him across the crowd at a recent community event and he couldn't stop staring at her, at how she looked now. If he left his other family and came to her and begged, she would never ever take him back.

Jennifer is about half the weight she was on that trip to Marineland a couple of years ago. She doesn't take any diabetes medication now. She still fights sugar cravings, and, when a craving gets out of hand, she takes a bite or two of a chocolate bar, chews reeeaaaallllyyy slowly, and throws the rest away.

Of all her old addictions that might come back, she's most afraid of the junk food addiction. Most afraid that one junk food meal will lead to another and then another and all that weight and unhealthiness will pile back on.

But most of the time she knows—she is in charge of her life. And it's so much better now, so much better, she ain't *never* goin' back to that way of living.

She'd like to see junk food restricted in Eeyou Istchee for everyone. Folks oughta know it isn't actually food.

Next up, she thinks, she might stop smoking. That'll probably be another tough one. And maybe she'll take up some other kinds of exercise. Like some of those weight or resistance exercises that sculpt your arms and ass. Years ago, she had a Christmas tree ass and everyone knew. It'd be good to have a famous ass again. A healthy, well-shaped, look-how-strong-I-am, famous ass.

15

The Story of Christopher Merriman of Eastmain

CHRISTOPHER Merriman was born on a farm in England about eight miles from Stratford-upon-Avon, the town where William Shakespeare was born. He grew up there during and just after World War II. With a population of a thousand, the town had four pubs and three hotels, and sometimes the town hall screened picture shows for ten pence a person. The picture show played at the front of the hall as adults sat on chairs and children sat on the floor and watched.

Christopher finished elementary school and then took an exam hoping to be accepted to grammar school, a type of specialized high school in England. That year, there were spaces in grammar school for only the top three students in the area. After writing the exam, Christopher placed fourth: it seemed that he would continue his schooling in the regular school until he was fifteen years of age. And then he would probably enter the work force, perhaps on the family farm.

Just then, the girl who placed third learned that her family was too poor to buy her grammar school uniform and without it she would be unable to attend. It was terrible news. And it meant that a place opened up for Christopher. But Christopher's parents were poor too, and they doubted that grammar school could be worth the money. The Catholic Sister heard about this and came to their house. Christopher's mother made a pot of tea, and they sat down together around the wooden table in the farmhouse kitchen. Gently and thoroughly, the Sister persuaded Christopher's parents that it would be wiser in the long run to educate him. He might make a good farmer, yes, but he had an opportunity now for schooling, an opportunity many kids in those days didn't get. It would do them all proud if he could learn to do other things too. And so Christopher went to grammar school in a town nearby.

For the most part, Christopher liked grammar school. He had friends and access to books, and he learned about everything from literature to mathematics to geology to biology. From time to time a teacher would make the students sit and listen to classical music on the radio. These sessions Christopher and his friends found mind-numbingly dull. They would stay awake by tapping out conversations in Morse code on each other's legs. Conversations about girls, about airplanes, about the cars they wanted to drive or pranks they wanted to play or lands they wanted to visit or homework they wanted not to do, about anything *except* classical music. And with that the music sessions became tolerable.

Some evenings, for something to do, he and his friends took the bus to the Royal Shakespeare Theatre in Stratford and watched a play performed by the Royal Shakespeare Company. The last bus back left before the play finished, so the boys would always stay until the end and walk back to their school. Tourists thought of Stratford-upon-Avon as an extraordinary place to which they would travel from far away, just to set their feet upon the cobblestones once walked by England's most famous writer, or to watch a play in the celebrated Royal Shakespeare Theatre. But to Christopher and his friends, it was just home, and, even with grammar school and theater, home could be a little dull.

World War II had ended in 1945 when Christopher was a six-year-old boy, and it had changed the country dramatically. Rural England did not recover for a long time. Christopher's childhood and teen years were years of people making do with what little they had. Sugar was rationed, so the kids in those years grew up without many treats. In fact, they could buy no candy in the whole of England until six years after the end of the war. If a girl in the village was about to marry, her friends and family gave her their clothing ration coupons and mended their own clothes to last another year, so that she could buy the fabric she needed to make a wedding dress.

Unfortunately, when Christopher graduated from grammar school, the economy was still struggling. It seemed there were no jobs available in England. Around that time, Christopher's biology teacher sailed across the ocean to the faraway city of Montréal to teach. From 1957 to 1960, he and Christopher corresponded by mail. "Canada is the country for you," the teacher wrote, when he heard that the employment situation in England wasn't looking up. "There's plenty of work here for fellows willing to flex their muscles."

On the 8th of April, 1960, sponsored for accommodations by his biology teacher, Christopher embarked a ship headed for Montréal. After about a week of sailing, the ship stopped in Québec City for the night because the St. Lawrence River was frozen, and immigration processing was done right there. The following day, they sailed again for Montréal. Right away, Christopher found work as a nighttime ambulance orderly at the Royal Victoria Hospital in Montréal. It was a job and it paid. The city was a bit much, though. Noisy and crowded. A young man could hardly breathe there, let alone stretch his legs.

After just a few weeks as an ambulance orderly, Christopher heard from his sponsor that a company called Hudson's Bay, or HBC, was hiring. His sponsor telephoned them, they sent an application to his apartment, and Christopher filled it out.

The HBC, it turned out, had trading posts all through the North in wilderness country, far from the city. They had work for Christopher in a trading post on a small island up at the top of James Bay, in the vast traditional land of the James Bay Cree, a territory several times the size of England.

It sounded wonderful.

Christopher boarded a train in Montréal as it chugged through big cities, and then through small towns and farmland not too different from the farmland of his own home, and then through mile after mile after of trees and rock and wilderness. After a two-day journey, the train finally arrived in the small town of Moosonee. There, Christopher boarded a single-engine Otter seaplane that flew him the rest of the way, landing on James Bay by the shore of Fort George island.

At Fort George, Christopher found no airports, hotels, arenas, gyms, or theatres. He saw no buses, ambulances, trains, or glaring city lights. What he did find was mosquitoes. Hordes of them. So many mosquitoes that an hour after he set foot in Fort George someone had to take him to the clinic because his face had so many bites it had swollen into something nearly unrecognizable. At the clinic, they gave him some medication that brought down the swelling and let him get to work.

The work waiting for Christopher kept him active with hauling supplies in and out of the warehouse. And the community of Indigenous people who lived there were generous and laughed easily. They gathered in bushland communities of cabins and teepees in the summer and moved further into the bush to their traplines and traditional land in winter. They used outdoor toilets and kerosene lamps and stoves that burned wood for heat, and they did a great deal of hunting and fishing. It wasn't altogether different from what Christopher had grown up with on the farm eight miles outside of Stratford-upon-Avon, but it was infinitely more interesting. It suited him just fine. He even grew accustomed to the mosquitoes, learning not to swat at them for the swatting only attracted them, and they no longer bothered him.

Life for the James Bay Cree was hard work. To stay alive in the sub-arctic, they moved nearly every waking minute: hunting on foot for food, cleaning and butchering and preserving game, chopping wood and hauling water, and putting up and taking down teepees. They didn't have or need many possessions.

Nor did they have much in the way of processed foods. Their diet was mostly what British folks called country meats: wild game like moose and caribou and grouse and beaver and muskrat and bear. Every now and again, one of the fellows from Austin Airlines, the main regional airline in those days, overnighted at the trading post with Christopher and, when he did, he brought him a steak or roast of beef from Moosonee. But most of the time, the trading post workers ate country meats provided by the HBC, or goose and fish they had hunted or caught themselves.

The Cree had a way to preserve goose meat so they could safely eat it through the winter months. They cooked and smoked it slowly in their teepees. The process dehydrated the meat into something like jerky and made for an intensely flavourful and very tough meat. You needed strong teeth to chew it and, if you ate too much of it, your jaw would threaten to fall off. It didn't take long at all for Christopher to develop a taste for the strong wild meats, smoked or not.

Behind the trading post, HBC had provided a small ice house. In winter, ice blocks would be cut from the frozen river and immersed in several feet of sawdust for insulation. Slowly, through the summer months, the blocks melted, but they stayed frozen long enough to keep Christopher's perishables cold and safe to eat until the onset of frost in fall, when the river would begin again to freeze. In 1965, the HBC sent him a kerosene refrigerator: a wick of burning kerosene heated the coils in the back of the frig, and the heat differential from that cooled the insulated chamber. But even with the luxuries of refrigeration, Christopher still often reached for smoked meats and their intense wild flavour.

Once every summer, a doctor visited the coastal communities by boat. He checked over every single person in each community, no matter how old or young, looking especially for signs of communicable diseases like tuberculosis and meningitis. Eventually, he brought with him an x-ray machine and x-ray technician. With the machine he could diagnose tuberculosis much earlier, before it caused permanent lung damage.

Along with the doctor came a dentist who extracted all teeth that were causing pain—there were never very many of them. The smoked goose the Cree ate kept their teeth and jaws strong, and the people didn't eat much sugar in those days, so teeth didn't easily decay. One year, the dentist came with a foot-operated drill. Fewer teeth had to be extracted then, as he drilled out the decay in a tooth and plugged the hole with a mercury filling.

As a general rule, there was no optician in the medical group and the doctor didn't usually check people's eyesight. Not very many people needed glasses, and, anyway, glasses weren't available that far north. If you lost your vision, you either travelled south for eye tests and spectacles, or you bumped into things and hoped that what you had bumped into wasn't a bear.

The medical team usually stayed in a community for a week or two. During the other fifty weeks of the year, if people needed medical attention, they used either the well-stocked medicine cabinet at the Hudson's Bay post—it held aspirin and laxatives and other over-the-counter remedies—or the ample traditional medical knowledge of healers in the community. Even though many people smoked unfiltered, hand-rolled cigarettes, they had little trouble warding off disease. Cancer and diabetes rarely bothered anyone.

But things were beginning to change. When Christopher arrived in Fort George, the HBC post had just switched from Morse code communications to radio, and a brand new microphone awaited him at his desk. Part of his job was to contact Austin Airways in Moose Factory twice a day. They flew to Fort George every week in small Beaver or Cessna planes and needed him to tell them about temperature and wind speeds and whether the whitecaps made it unsafe for their aircraft to land. He also took down any telegrams or medical information from the hospital in Moose Factory to be passed on to people in Fort George who had family in the hospital. He ended his radio conversations with "Over and out."

In the early years, Christopher's Gloucestershire accent was so thick that the Austin Airways operator in Moose Factory couldn't understand him at all, and Christopher had to summon his manager to talk to the Moose Factory operator instead. His manager was from Scotland and had an Aberdeen accent every bit as difficult to understand as Christopher's accent and, when either of them spoke into the microphone, the airwaves of Northern Québec might have been mistaken for those of the United Kingdom. (The poor Moose Factory operator couldn't understand a word and openly longed for the old Morse Code where accents hadn't mattered.)

For a while, Christopher worked for the Hudson's Bay Company in Fort George, and then he was posted to Waskaganish (or Rupert's House as the HBC people called it), then to Fort Albany across the bay, and that was the end of the two-year term. Christopher sailed back to England for a vacation and half-expected to do as many HBC men did after two years in James Bay: find another post further west. But upon returning to Montréal after his vacation, he signed up for another two-year term. It wasn't likely that any other job would suit him half as well as the one in James Bay.

In 1962, he was posted to Eastmain (where a girl named Emily Gilpin was housekeeper) and then to Whapmagoostui (or

Great Whale as the HBC folks said), and then to Fort George and Waskaganish. In 1963, he worked in Nemaska, and from 1964 to 1967, he was back in Eastmain. When he arrived for a second time in Eastmain, the housekeeper Emily Gilpin was in Nova Scotia. She returned to Eastmain after her contract finished, and Christopher approached her and asked if she might agree to be his housekeeper once more. One thing led to another and, when he was posted to Fort Albany in 1967, Emily followed him. They were married in the residential school there, and in 1973, their son came along.

In 1979, after twelve years in Fort Albany, they were posted back to Eastmain. It was a tiny community then, just sixteen two-bedroom houses, but each house held three or four families. As often as they could, people headed to the bush where they could live more comfortably with unlimited space and more privacy than the houses in town allowed.

Years later, in 1991, the HBC posts in James Bay were taken over by the Northern Company, and Christopher had the opportunity to go to Moose Factory. He asked Emily if she wanted to go.

"I'm home now," she said, "I think I don't want to leave."

So they settled in Eastmain with their son, and it became Christopher's home.

And still, the changes came. In the late '70s and early '80s, Austin Airways stopped flying north, and Air Creebec took on their mantle with planes that could carry more people and cargo than the Cessnas and Beavers of Austin Airways had carried. Radio communications changed too, and the "Over and out" fell away like other outmoded expressions. Telephone lines were laid all across the region, but were soon followed by cell phones and satellite phones that bypassed landlines altogether.

The biggest upheaval of all came when the James Bay Hydroelectric Project transformed the landscape to generate hydro for the Province of Québec to sell (mostly to United States).

Anticipating that the waterways of Eeyou Istchee would be significantly altered by the Project, the Province of Québec told the people of Nemaska that they had to relocate, partly because the Project would divert the river in a way that might flood their homes, and partly because Hudson's Bay Company was closing the Nemaska post. Similarly, the Province told the people of Fort George Island, where Christopher had first worked, that the diversions would affect their island and they had to choose whether to erect huge barriers in the water to protect the island from the increased force of the diverted river, or to relocate the entire town to Chisasibi. They held a referendum and voted to move the town, though the move meant quite a bit of money for some people and huge losses for others. In the long run, both relocations caused hard feelings. The people of Eastmain, however, were never told all of the ways a diverted waterway would affect them. The day the new Hydroelectric Project began running was the day the Eastmain River, which carried fresh water in the direction of James Bay, was reduced by ninety percent. That reduction allowed the saltwater from the James Bay tides to course fifteen kilometres upriver, turning Eastmain's drinking and cooking water to salt.

The Eastmain people had expected a reduction in river flow, but they were stunned by the ways in which it turned their water brackish. The upheaval was massive. The plants and fish in the river died. The water itself was undrinkable and people had to melt snow, have water trucked in, hike to local springs, or drive long distances to buy it bottled. Eventually Hydro-Québec built a multi-million-dollar water-treatment plant, one of the most sophisticated in the country, so that people in the area could have drinking water.

The community received some compensation for the mayhem the Project had caused and spent it on a new fire hall, medical centre, arena, and gymnasium. With all the construction came roads for the big construction machines. And with the roads came more movement from the community to Val-d'Or and Radisson and Chibougamau. And with the increased movement came a good deal more liquor, much of it brought in by the workers on the Project. Even youth now had easier access to alcohol. The traditional ways of life began quickly to fall away.

In time, the river plants and fish were replaced by plants and fish that could survive in saltwater, and in time the people were able again to bring back some of the traditional ways. But by then, many people had stopped hunting and fishing and instead purchased their groceries at the store or drove into one of the towns for Kentucky Fried Chicken. It became a common thing to hear about children, who had grown up on pork chops and sliced meat and soft drinks, who refused to eat goose or fish or traditional food at all. Even life in the bush camps, outside of town, changed and people began hauling generators and sometimes even computers and televisions out to their camps.

Christopher grieved many of these changes and the destruction they wrought onto a place and a way of life he had come to love. But his wife Emily just shook her head at each one and smiled a little smile: "That's life, Christopher," she would say. "Change is life."

Things were changing in England too. Christopher's parents aged. In his mother's last months, she would waken in the mornings and say to Christopher's sister, "I'm still here, dear. I haven't died yet." But one morning, while Christopher was in Canada, she didn't make her usual announcement, and didn't waken. Not long after, his father, from whom Christopher had inherited his love of independence, also began to wane. Christopher boarded a plane then to see him one last time, but he passed away while Christopher was en route.

In 1980, Christopher flew back to England for his biennial visit with his remaining family. While he was there, his sister told him to go to get checked for diabetes. "It runs in the family," she said. "Half of your relatives have it. You should at least know if you have it too." He had no symptoms, but the next time Christopher went to the clinic for something, he asked the medical team to check his blood sugar. And there it was: diabetes.

To cope with this new condition, Christopher had to make a few changes in his routine. He had to check his blood sugar when he woke in the morning and he had to watch carefully what he ate. They were easy changes to make and became habit soon enough. His diet centred upon fresh healthy food. Emily was an excellent cook and baker, and her family hunted and kept them well-supplied with game. And his lifestyle already had a great deal of activity in it as he transferred supplies from planes or boats to trucks, from trucks to warehouses, and from warehouses to store shelves. Diabetes management just became part of his life, like getting up in the morning and going to bed at night.

After a few years, the doctor said it was time for him to start taking pills every day at noon and at dinner. And four years after that, Christopher got food poisoning and was sent to the Chisasibi hospital to recover. There, the doctor noticed that his blood sugar was dangerously high, even though he was taking his pills regularly. So they hooked him up to an IV to bring it down, and they also gave him insulin for the first time. From now on, he was going to have inject himself with insulin a few times a day, the doctor said, and he would have to stay in the hospital until he learned how to do it. A nurse patiently showed him how to fill the syringe and push it into the fat below his skin, and she made him practise poking the needle into an orange. When he had the confidence to inject himself into his stomach, he could go home to Eastmain.

Injecting himself regularly with insulin and looking after his diabetes became a natural part of life. Eventually, Christopher was awarded a certificate from the Cree Board of Health for the ways he successfully managed his diabetes. He managed it so well that most people around him didn't even know he was diabetic.

Emily's health was much more of a family concern. When she was young, she had contracted tuberculosis. As a result, she had limited use of her lungs. She had spent some time in a sanatorium in Hamilton in her teen years to strengthen her lungs, but was nevertheless susceptible to pneumonia and collapse. In the last seven years of her life, the weakness set in again and her breathing became difficult. They had a compressor at home, a machine that helped her breathe. Every day, when Christopher came home from work, he would immediately check that the compressor was working properly and that it had enough water. Still, two or three times a year, Emily would have breathing troubles and they would have to rush her into the clinic and the clinic would med-evac her to Val-d'Or. In her later years, as her lungs weakened further, she had quite a few surgeries, and with each one she said to Christopher, "Well, that's life."

Once, she was rushed to the Chibougamau hospital, and the family continued to visit her there for the next weeks. When they inquired at Cree Patient Services for details about when she would be discharged, they found that CPS had lost track of her for two weeks, and hadn't known where she was. All the while, she had been well looked after in Chibougamau and had no idea she was lost. When the whole story came out, she laughed along with everyone else, and said, as she often did, "Well, that's life too."

After one particularly bad bout of pneumonia in 2013, the hospital in Val-d'Or called Christopher to pick her up and bring her home. When he arrived, he could see that Emily clearly wasn't strong enough to board a plane, and then disembark in Waskaganish as it refueled, board it again, and so forth. She didn't have strength enough for the trip. The doctor and nurse agreed, so Christopher stayed in Val-d'Or with Emily. Her breathing worsened, and two days later she passed away. "That's life," she would have said, but she was no longer there to say it.

When Christopher returned home, the house was strangely silent, and he, who had spent so much time listening for the sound of the compressor, caught himself listening for it still. Or walking into their bedroom out of habit to make sure the machine had enough water in it. Or hearing her voice as he moved through the house he had shared with her all those years.

Christopher Merriman is 78 years old. If he had stayed in England, in Shakespeare's town, he would have grown up just another British bloke. Instead, he has lived with the James Bay Cree for 58 wonderful years and has had a life much richer than anything he imagined as a boy. He long ago retired from HBC and took up work with the Cree Government in Land Registry to keep himself busy and out of trouble. He's a decade and a half past his "use by" date, as he says, and he reminds the Chief and Council of Eastmain that they ought to feel free to replace him if they have someone younger who needs the job. He's ready to step aside and train someone else if necessary.

And the changes keep coming. When his grandkids go trick-or-treating on Hallowe'en, they each collect entire pillowcases full of candy, more candy than all the children in the whole of England would have had when Christopher was a boy. His grandkids bought Christopher a tablet and Skype with him when they can. When Christopher first arrived in Eastmain, "Skype" wasn't even a word.

With each new change, he thinks of Emily: "That's life, Christopher," she would have said. "That's life."

16

The Story of Jennifer Susan Annistin* of Waskaganish

JENNIFER Susan Annistin of Waskaganish was a good wife and mother. She lived with her husband and three kids. During the days she worked, and then she came home in the evenings and looked after her family. She cooked dinner, she prepared lunches, she got everything ready for breakfast the next morning, and she hauled out the trash and all of her husband's empty beer cans. She helped the kids with their homework or whatever they needed. Every couple of days, she did the laundry for everyone in the house, she washed the floors and vacuumed, scrubbed the bathrooms, and cleaned the frig. She went to her kids' sport or school events and arranged family evenings with friends and weekends out in the bush. Everything that had to happen in that house, Jennifer did it. It was exhausting and she didn't enjoy all of it, but as long as she did all those things, she knew she was a good wife and mother.

In 2002, Jennifer did a 300-kilometre walk to experience what her ancestors had experienced in their long-distance treks. At the end of it, she felt sore all over and her feet ached more than they ever had before, but she also felt strong and capable of anything. Her mind was at ease. She did the walk again in 2003 and in 2004.

*Names and details in this story have been changed to protect identities.

In 2006, Jennifer was tired all the time. Tired and anxious and *off*. Maybe she was going through a bout of depression. Or maybe it was diabetes. Diabetes ran in her family.

"Go to the clinic," her sister said. "If it's something like high blood pressure, you'll just need a pill and you'll feel better."

Jennifer went to the clinic. The doctor took some blood and sent her home. Soon after, the clinic called her back and told her to come in right away. They had the results from her blood test and it was urgent.

She went back to the clinic, and slumped down in the chair in the exam room. She had never been so tired.

The doctor came in and closed the door behind him.

"Have you ever heard anything about anyone in your family having cancer?" he asked.

Jennifer thought for a while. Then she remembered her uncle. He had had leukemia, a cancer of the blood. They gave him a bone marrow transplant and that got rid of his cancer and they sent him home to recover. When he stepped off the plane at home, his community held a feast to celebrate his homecoming and the end of his cancer. There was plenty of food—moose and beaver and fish—and everyone in the whole community came up to him and gave him a big hug or shook his hand. He was a popular guy and people were happy to see him and to know he had that cancer licked. But someone who shook his hand or hugged him had a cold and passed it on to him. His cancer was gone, but his immune system wasn't very strong yet: the cold developed into a bad case of pneumonia and he died a couple of weeks after that feast.

Jennifer told all of this to the doctor, and then yawned. He listened thoughtfully.

"I, uh, I think you might have leukemia too," he said. "We're going to send you to Montréal—you might even get the same specialist your uncle had. But there are better medications and treatments for leukemia now than there were when he was sick. And in fact, we're going to start you on some of those medications now, before we even have all the test results back. The trick to beating leukemia, if that's what this is, is getting it in the early stages."

Jennifer started the medication. A week later the test results came back. She had exactly the same leukemia that her uncle had had. Other than exhaustion, she had felt no symptoms at all.

Jennifer's mom heard "leukemia" and thought her daughter was about to die, and cried herself to pieces. But Jennifer herself was so surprised that she just went about her days as if nothing had happened. By now she was weak and couldn't even do something as simple as wash the dishes, so her mother washed the dishes for her, and cried while she did them.

One evening Jennifer sat down and watched a movie in which the actor Mandy Moore played a girl with leukemia. While she watched the girl on screen go through the things that she was going to go through, a fountain of sadness began flowing inside of Jennifer. Sadness for her uncle who had died, sadness for herself because she might die now too, and sadness for the people who would miss her. She began to weep.

And then it was time to go to Montréal.

In Montréal, the doctors saw right away that Jennifer was very sick. They were surprised she was walking at all. But Jennifer had felt like this for a long time already and barely noticed their expressions of shock and concern.

The oncologist, a doctor specializing in the treatment of cancer, gave her chemotherapy pills that would gradually kill the cancer in her blood. "This is something new," she said. "I wish I'd had this pill for your uncle because it would have helped him."

The treatment began working right away and that was good news. It meant that Jennifer would not need a bone marrow transplant like her uncle had had. She could even go home and take the pills every day there.

The oncologist wanted to see her each month. The problem was that Jennifer lived way up in Waskaganish. Flying down and back once a month on the Waskaganish-Nemaska-Chibougamau-Montréal milk run wasn't reasonable. A single doctor's appointment would take three days, more if the weather was bad. They decided together that her home clinic would take her blood every month and send it to the cancer clinic laboratory in Montréal where they would run a special test that detects even the smallest amount of cancer. Every third month, Jennifer would fly down and visit the oncologist in person. And every single day, without exception, she would take her chemotherapy pills. They were as important to her, the oncologist said, as insulin is to someone with severe diabetes.

Jennifer expected to get side effects from the chemotherapy. She met other people on the same treatment who had terrible nausea and spent time each day hung over the toilet bowl, vomiting. And their hair either fell out or lost its lustre and dried into something like straw. But Jennifer had no side effects at all.

Gradually, the cancer in Jennifer's blood was going away. For a while, life became less terrifying. Then, early in 2007, she began to menstruate more than she had ever menstruated before—and she had always had troubles with heavy menstruation.

A few months later, the doctors decided to insert a specific type of IUD (intra-uterine contraceptive device) into her uterus, thinking that it might slow or minimize her monthly blood loss. She would still bleed heavily for a little while from hormonal fluctu-ations, they said, but then the bleeding would correct itself.

It didn't correct itself. Jennifer bled more than she had ever bled. She bled so much that the IUD passed right out of her in one of the giant clots of blood that were always coming out of her these days—and she didn't even notice it had happened until the gynecologist gave her a CT scan and discovered the device was no longer in her uterus. Usually, an IUD exiting the uterus is very painful, but Jennifer hadn't felt a thing.

And still she was bleeding. Instead of menstruating for a few days of each month, like most women do, Jennifer bled every single day for months and months and months.

In November, she visited a new doctor in the Waskaganish clinic. The doctor noted Jennifer's excessive menstruation and prescribed some pills to stop the bleeding. Jennifer talked about her leukemia and the chemotherapy medication she was taking—but the doctor didn't seem to pay attention and said again that these new pills should stop the bleeding.

Jennifer started taking the pills.

And everything got so much worse. She bled and bled and bled, more than she ever had. So much blood flowed now that she could feel it squish between her legs every time she moved. In just two days, she was white from loss of blood.

Her sister came to her house that Saturday on her way to work. "What's wrong with you?" she asked. "You're so white you don't even look Cree anymore."

"I'm having my period and the doctor put me on these pills and they're not helping."

"Call the clinic," she said. "You of all people can't mess around with this stuff."

"It's Saturday. The clinic is closed."

"Call. There's always a nurse on call. Call the clinic."

Her sister left for work and Jennifer called the nurse. The nurse knew she was a cancer patient and told her to meet him there in thirty minutes.

With each passing minute, Jennifer felt worse. Her heartbeat was weak and fluttery and she couldn't get enough air. She had a bit of laundry to do in the thirty minutes before her meeting at the clinic and stumbled downstairs to the laundry room. But when she got there, she slumped against the washing machine. She didn't have strength even to sort laundry. She felt as if she might die in the next couple of minutes. Maybe it was her time. But if it was—she certainly didn't want to die in her laundry room.

She gathered all her strength and started the long journey upstairs, leaning heavily on the rail to pull herself up. It was every bit as difficult as the 300 kilometres she had walked years back.

When she got upstairs, her twenty-year-old son was there.

"I'm getting dressed to go to the clinic," she said. "If something happens to me in the next few minutes, call the clinic. I don't know if I can make it there."

Her son looked at her and nodded wordlessly.

She was too weak to drive, she realized. Her sister was at work, her husband was out drinking, her parents were in the bush, and her son didn't have his driver's license. She was alone. She called her pastor and he came around and took her to the clinic.

The nurse at the clinic was shocked at the state of her and quickly arranged to med-evac her down to Val-d'Or.

In Val-d'Or, the gynecologist met her, also shocked. "You need a blood transfusion!" she said. "Your body is almost out of blood! What happened?"

Jennifer explained how she'd been bleeding for months—and the gynecologist interrupted: "You're a cancer patient! With blood cancer!" she said. "Why didn't they send you here right away?"

"There's a new doctor at home. I don't think she even read my file. I told her I was bleeding and she prescribed the pills. Then I talked about leukemia and chemotherapy, but she didn't seem to hear me. She just said the pills would make me stop bleeding over the weekend. I think they made me bleed more."

The gynecologist looked at the pills the Waskaganish doctor had prescribed.

"Of course you're bleeding," she said. "These pills should never be taken by someone on chemotherapy! The doctor should have known that. And—how can a doctor *not read* a patient file??"

"Well," Jennifer said, "now I'm here. I thought I was going to die so this is better."

And then she fell asleep.

The gynecologist gave Jennifer a blood transfusion and did a process called dilation and curettage (D&C), where the uterus is cleaned out, and gave her iron pills to rebuild her blood supply.

Jennifer had lost a massive amount of blood. If it had taken much longer for her to get to Val-d'Or, she would have bled to death. The gynecologist began to wonder if the chemotherapy wasn't making the bleeding worse. Jennifer reminded her that she had had problems with bleeding earlier in her life, before the chemotherapy, but still, the gynecologist was suspicious—and prevented Jennifer from taking the chemotherapy pills.

Jennifer began to feel a bit panicky then. The chemo was saving her life. Her oncologist had warned that she must never miss a day of chemotherapy because her cancer could quickly come back, worse than before, and she would have no hope.

Finally, she convinced the gynecologist at least to call the oncologist and talk about it.

And over the phone, the oncologist shouted exactly what Jennifer had said: "Ms. Annistin had problems with bleeding long before she had cancer! Obviously, her bleeding is *not* being caused by the chemo pills—and in fact they're saving her life. Will you please get her back on those pills?!!"

The gynecologist relented. After four days without chemotherapy, Jennifer began taking her chemo pills again.

Two other things happened then: the gynecologist ran a whole bunch of tests on Jennifer. It turned out that she had a condition called adenomyosis and it had caused all the heavy bleeding.

And she also gave Jennifer a note to put in her Waskaganish medical file: "URGENT: If Jennifer ever menstruates abnormally or haemorrhages in any way, or has unusual symptoms of any sort, send her straight to the gynecologist in Val-d'Or."

With the new treatments, Jennifer's bleeding slowly lessened though she still bled more than she was supposed to. And slowly the cancer in her blood began to disappear. Each cancer screen looked better than the one before, until the screens came back cancer-free.

Later her son said, "Remember that time you almost didn't make it to the clinic? You looked so sick I was afraid for you! I'm glad you're okay now."

Jennifer *was* okay—but she made a few changes at home. Even when she had been at death's door, her family had expected her to do all the housework. She could have died doing laundry. What a way to go.

"From now on," she announced to her family, "I'm not doing anyone's personal laundry. I'm doing my own laundry and the towels for the house. If the rest of you want clean clothes, you can wash them. If you don't want to do laundry, then wear dirty clothes."

She would always remember 2007 as the year of the haemorrhaging.

For a few beautiful months, Jennifer felt normal. She had normal levels of iron in her blood, she had normal amounts of blood, and she had normal cancer-free blood. She still bled too much, all the time, but it was at a level she could cope with.

Then she went to the doctor for a routine check-up and found out that she had diabetes. The doctor gave her some pills. So much for normal. *Whatever*, she thought. *After cancer and haemorrhaging, diabetes isn't scary at all.* Other than taking her pills regularly, she didn't pay much attention to the new diagnosis.

In 2008, Jennifer sat down and wrote a letter to the corporate sector of Waskaganish saying that she needed her own place. She didn't write a word about her health problems—not the bleeding, not the leukemia, not the diabetes. A friend read the application before she sent it in.

"Jennifer," she said, "maybe you should tell them about your health problems. Tell them the cancer might come back and how hard it is to deal with. Tell them that you need your own space if you're going to be healthy. Be honest."

It wasn't a comfortable thing to write. Jennifer didn't want to think of herself as a person with more needs than other people. She didn't like speaking badly of anyone, even if it was just that her husband wasn't there for her when she needed help, or that in their home no one looked after her when she was sick. She didn't want people to pity her, she didn't like to sound like she was complaining, and she especially didn't want to think of herself as someone who would turn her back on a marriage. Writing those things made her feel guilty.

But in the end, she took her friend's advice and re-wrote the application. She wrote frankly about her year of cancer and about her year of haemorrhaging and how she needed space and time to herself for healing. She wrote that her cancer might come back, and, if it did, she would need reliable people around and a home where she didn't have to worry about running a complicated household or about the troubles surrounding a husband who hadn't yet confronted his addictions. Her doctor in Waskaganish also wrote a letter of support, and a nurse who knew Jennifer's background talked to her and showed her that moving to her own home to look after herself was the right thing to do. Her friends and parents supported her, her kids were grown and didn't need her at home anymore, her son said he just wanted her to be happy and knew his dad had no plans to stop drinking. Even her pastor supported her decision.

At first the council was reluctant to give her housing: they thought that she and her husband were just squabbling like any long-married couple, would soon mend their relationship, and she would want to stay where she was. But they changed their minds and one day she received a letter that a house was being built for her. In 2010, she could move in.

Jennifer spoke to her husband then, gave him two years to clean up his act, and said she would leave if he didn't. He tried, for a while. But addictions are powerful and his drinking won out again. In 2010, Jennifer left his house and moved into her own place.

As she was out shopping, buying her own pots and pans and towels and sheets, she thought about guilt. Once, she had believed that two married people have to stick together no matter what. Once, she had believed that good moms didn't have their own lives: everything they did was for their families. They would put up with anything at all from their families and would do everything possible to make them look good. Once, she would have been wracked with guilt just for thinking about looking after herself. Cancer had changed all of that. She had to look after herself. No one else was going to do it. She knew that now. It was a good change.

When she moved into her own place, she felt neither guilt over her choice nor anger with anyone. Only peace. Plenty of peace.

Jennifer loved her new home, and her health began to improve noticeably now that, for the first time in her adult life, she could focus on herself. Her granddaughter moved in with her to keep her company, she still had plenty of contact with her kids and other grandkids, and she was able to be more involved in the community. The cancer stayed where it belonged (in remission and not in her body) and she didn't pay too much attention to the diabetes. But still, she was bleeding. She had been menstruating non-stop now for about five years. It was inconvenient, expensive, and annoying. And kind of amazing that a person could bleed for that long and not die.

In March of 2012, without warning, it began to storm—and Jennifer began haemorrhaging again. Outside snow fell by the bucket, and inside it felt like blood was pouring out of her by the bucket. This time, she didn't hesitate. She went straight to the clinic.

The doctor there called the gynecologist in Val-d'Or, and explained what was happening. Then she turned to Jennifer.

"They want you in Val-d'Or right away."

They both looked out the window. The storm was getting worse. Snowdrifts were piling up under the clinic windows and cars on the road had slowed to a crawl.

Still, Jennifer went to the airport. The winds were too strong for planes to land, the airline worker said. There would be no flights today.

Jennifer called the clinic. "I'm going to have to drive there," she said.

"The weather's insane! You can't drive."

"If I wait, I'm either gonna go into shock or lose so much blood I might die—you know this. It's less risky for me to drive. I have to take care of myself. I'll call you when I get there."

She called her ex then and he offered to drive her to Val-d'Or so she wouldn't have to go alone.

Now she hurried. Her ex fueled up the car, she grabbed an armful of extra pads to absorb the blood flowing out of her, and they drove as quickly as the roads allowed from Waskaganish all the way down to Val-d'Or. In the storm, the trip took two hours longer than it usually would, and by the time she got there, she had that old familiar weakness from loss of blood.

In Val-d'Or they were waiting for her. They had scheduled her surgery a few days later, but, when they saw her, they gave her papers to sign and wheeled her into surgery right away. Jennifer didn't even have time to call the clinic in Waskaganish and tell them what was happening.

Again the surgeon did the D&C procedure and everything worked out nicely. They gave her a hormone injection to help control the bleeding, and said she would have to get one of these injections every three months. When her strength came back again, Jennifer and her ex drove back home.

At first, it seemed like the shots weren't doing anything, but then Jennifer started bleeding less and less, until her menstrual cycle finally, after all those years, became normal again.

The time had come for Jennifer to focus on her diabetes. For a long time, her other health problems had seemed so much more pressing that she hadn't given it much thought. But then a doctor told her that diabetes is as lethal as cancer. If she didn't take it seriously, it would finish the job that cancer started. After all the effort she had put into building a healthy life for herself, a life where she mattered, it didn't make sense to ignore diabetes.

She was already eating carefully to help her body fight the cancer and the bleeding, but she met with a nutritionist nonetheless, and made a few more changes in her diet. She also began to measure her blood sugar levels regularly and to take insulin.

The doctor said she should walk. That was a bit frightening. When she had been so sick with cancer or haemorrhaging, she had forced herself into physical activity and had collapsed from exhaustion. Still, she gave walking a thirty-minute try.

It felt okay. Good even. It reminded her of those long long walks she had done ten years earlier. Maybe she would work up to one of them again.

It had been a long journey and a difficult decade. And what she had learned most of all was that the key to good health—physical and emotional and spiritual—was looking after herself with as much care and diligence as she had once looked after others. For the people who loved her and wanted her to stick around, it was the most important thing she could do.

Stories We Heard Along the Way: Dogs

We heard many stories about dogs. One of the things storytellers said was that the health of a community is reflected in the health of the dogs: a healthy community had well-treated healthy dogs and an unhealthy community didn't. They spoke also of being able to tell something about a person by how s/he treats dogs. People who treat dogs well are likely to treat their families well too, they said. Some of the storytellers in this book spoke of seeing ill-treated dogs as a source of extreme stress. They are deeply bothered, they said, when they see a dog that is starving or too thin, a dog that is always tied up and cannot get enough exercise, a short-haired dog left outside in winter, or a chained-up dog without plenty of water within reach. It reminded them, they said, of being trapped in residential school when they didn't always have enough food or water or exercise or warm clothing.

•

From time to time, some Public Health and Safety workers used unconventional ways of fundraising: they would drive to someone's house in the daytime while the owner was at work, untie a dog that was tied up there, and take it to the pound. The owner would then have to drive to the pound and pay a 250-dollar fee to get the dog back.

•

Before the days of snowmobiles, dogs were essential to lives of the James Bay Cree. They were especially necessary for travel over long distances and for travel on ice or checking fishnets in winter. The dogs could sense where the ice was thin and would avoid it to run on thicker ice instead. If there was a sudden change in the weight of what they were pulling because someone had fallen through the ice or something had fallen off the sled, the dogs would stop immediately until the situation could be remedied. Dog training was done without punishment. A young dog would be trained from the time it was small by tying it to a sled with other dogs who would teach it to pull properly. Soon enough, the dog would understand the commands and would know how to pull a sled. The difficult part of working with dogs was making sure their leads didn't tangle.

●

Thousands of years ago, dogs were natural hunters who hunted in packs like wolves. But dogs of today have been domesticated and they no longer have those instincts. If they are not fed, they usually cannot hunt nor find enough food to survive and will suffer a great deal before dying of starvation.

●

When the people lived entirely on the land, they would eat large game (like moose or caribou) from the inside out. The best part was what was inside the intestine—usually greens and lichen that were full of vitamins and had very strong flavours. After that had been eaten, the people would eat the innermost organs, and then the outer organs. Most of the meat (muscle) was fed to the dogs. In those days, Cree dogs were highly valued and very well treated even in the months when the dogs were not working or in the years after they were too old to work—partly because the people depended on dogs for hunting and travel, and partly because providing their dogs with enough food and water and exercise was part of showing respect to the Creator.

17

The Story of Raquel Emmeline Welsch* of Wemindji

THE MORNING sunshine slips into the bedroom through the blinds and Raquel opens her eyes and yawns. She reaches for the glucometer beside the bed, as she does every morning, pricks herself with the lancet, squeezes some blood onto a paper strip and slides it into the machine. This morning her blood sugar is 9. Not bad at all for someone who has had diabetes for as long as she has. But it's Tuesday, the day of her medical check-up, and no doubt the doc will find something to complain about. Ah, no big deal. Raquel will be grumpy for an hour and then laugh it off like she always does. Life is good. She tosses the strip and lancet in the trash, and dresses for her day.

At her last check-up, the doc went on about her nighttime munchies. She had been diligent all day of every day that whole month, and, yeah, sometimes at night she had given in. Sometimes at night, before she went to bed, the cutest little devil appeared on her right shoulder whispering, "C'mon Raquel, just a few chips. You know you really want 'em."

The devil was right, she really did want them.

*Names and details in this story have been changed to protect identities.

Mostly she ignored him, but sometimes she pulled out a small bowl—didn't wanna overdo it—and dumped a few chips in, plunked her butt on the sofa, and really savoured 'em, each one.

Of course the doc nagged: "No eating after eight," he said, again. "It's why you've been feeling so tired lately."

She shakes her head thinking of him. Doesn't he get it? She's been trying to stop the occasional night time munchies for ten years already. If she *coulda* done it, she *woulda* done it long ago, but that little devil is just too smart and too cute. Raquel isn't a big eater, so her blood sugar never goes too terribly high, and her health is in good shape for someone who's had diabetes for so long. Thirty years and nothing but a bit of laser surgery to clear up one eye— and that might not even have been the diabetes. It might just have been getting old. And what's the point of getting old if you're not gonna enjoy a few chips every now and then before you go to bed?

Raquel was born in Ontario, close to Thunder Bay, and grew up in Moosonee and Moose Factory. Her mom, who came from Attawapiskat, had lost her own mom at age 3 and had spent many years in residential school. Her teachers there said that people who spoke Cree were stupid, and, if she didn't want her own children to be stupid she would have to make sure they never spoke it. Raquel begged her mom to speak to her in Cree, but her mom never did.

"I want you to speak English," she would say.

Sometimes Raquel asked her about abuse in residential school.

"Oh, don't worry Raquel. I was never abused, it was okay," she said. And then she would start talking about throwing up spoiled food and being made to eat it anyways.

"But Mom," Raquel would say, "That's abuse!"

"Oh no, honey," her mom would say. "Abuse is sexual stuff. When they do those. . . sexual things. None of that happened to me."

Raquel's mom did her best with the ten kids she had, but she couldn't remember her own mom and didn't know how to be the greatest mom herself. She loved her kids, but could never show them affection or concern. She couldn't really say what she wanted from them, and so her kids were always guessing. She kept herself clean and brushed her teeth and trimmed her toenails, but she never taught these things to her children. Only when Raquel went to school did she learn that she should be doing those things herself; her mom had never mentioned them.

What her mom did talk about was bingo.

"I wanna play bingo! Find me money to go!" she would shout at Raquel's dad. And he would shout back that she could have bingo money after the cupboards were full and the frig had some food in it.

They sure were poor. Raquel had one pair of underwear and one pair of socks that she washed at night before she went to bed so that she had something clean to wear the next day, and if she didn't wash 'em, she had to wear 'em dirty, and so she always washed 'em. They lived on pasta and rice and bread sandwiches smeared with butter or, if there was no butter, with lard. Cheap foods. There were treats, though. Sometimes each kid got an apple—and with ten kids and two parents a dozen apples disappeared in about thirty seconds. If her dad went hunting and brought home a goose, each person could have a small piece of goose meat and as many dumplings in gravy as he or she wanted. Salad appeared on the dinner table on payday. And real milk was too expensive, but sometimes there would be a glass of powdered milk by each plate.

But Raquel didn't know she was poor until she went away to school where she met people who had more. She didn't feel poor. She didn't have many clothes but she had some. The foods they ate were cheap, but there was never a day, never a single day, where there weren't three meals on the table. Her mom and dad might not have been perfect, but they did okay. Her family had it better than some others.

Truth was, Raquel didn't need much food. She never was a big eater. Sometimes she even forgot to eat. Sometimes, as a kid, she would be running around and get the shakes so badly she could hardly stand.

"It's m' nerves again!" she would holler. "Bring me some juice!"

She gulped the juice and, in a few seconds, her nerves steadied right out. Later, after she learned the shakes were a sign of pre-diabetes or low blood sugar, she laughed until her belly shook that she had once believed juice was calming her "nerves" and not her blood sugar.

When she was five years old, Raquel was sent to residential school, but even there she counted herself lucky because she boarded with a lady from Ottawa who cared for her very well. Still, she was lonely and didn't want to go back. "Okay," her father said, "This family has had enough residential school. You're not going back."

Instead she went to school in Moosonee for a few years and then to a boarding high school in North Bay where she made friends from all around the world and even won a scholarship for her out-going personality. Raquel studied there until Grade 11. Then her dad got cancer and Raquel stayed home. She helped her mom look after the house and the kids, and she married a guy who had taken a shine to her.

Her mom still wasn't doing a whole lot of child-rearing, and someone had to do it, so Raquel did. She raised her younger brothers and sisters and taught them what she had learned. She made sure they cleaned themselves and ate properly and tidied up after them-selves and did their homework and got into college and were kind and compassionate and took responsibility for their own lives. She must have done okay because those kids all turned out pretty good.

Raquel liked raising kids so much she figured she may as well start in on her own. While she was still raising her siblings and just 18 years old, the year her dad died of cancer, Raquel had her first boy. And every second year after that, she had another baby boy until there were four of them running around.

Except for her first pregnancy, Raquel got gestational diabetes each time, and each time was worse than the time before.

With the last one, she spent almost three months in the hospital as the doctors watched her and her baby and worried.

"Raquel," the doctor finally said. "We have to tie your tubes. You can't have more kids. Your blood sugar is too erratic when you're pregnant—your body can't take it."

"No way," she said. "I still don't have a girl."

"You might want a girl," he said, "but I want you to live. And so does your husband. And so do your sons."

Raquel had her tubes tied then. She and her husband talked about adopting a girl. But the truth was that they couldn't afford more kids. And that doc was right. Her gestational diabetes WAS bad—in fact, it had become type 2 diabetes, the kind that never goes away. That wasn't much of a surprise. Nearly everyone in her whole huge family had type 2 diabetes. She had kind of been expecting it.

Raquel and her husband decided they would raise their kids in a different atmosphere than the one Raquel had grown up in. They didn't want to be shouting parents; they wanted to sit down and reason with their kids instead. But kids can drive a person crazy, and sometimes shouting was all Raquel wanted to do. So she talked to her aunts to understand her own mom and why she had been the way she had been. Once she heard more about her mom's life, Raquel understood why she had shouted and she also understood how not to shout at her own kids. Work took Raquel and her husband all over the place—North Bay, Whapmagoostui, Wemindji, and through all the moves and changes, she and her husband put effort into having a home where things got talked through and not shouted.

Raquel doesn't have to go to work today and there are a few hours yet before her check-up. Time enough to bake a cake. She sets the butter on the counter to soften, hauls up the bags of flour and sugar and cocoa, preheats the oven, and opens her cookbook. In every recipe in the book—bread, pies, biscuits, jam, cookies, cakes, casseroles, crackers, you name it—she long ago crossed out the original amount of sugar and wrote in a quarter or a third of what the recipe calls for. That way she can enjoy a bite or two of her own baking without spiking her sugar levels, and that way her family long ago got used to things being less sweet. Her kids never gorged on sweets the way she sees that sugar-addicted kids do. And even though her desserts have less sugar, they always have more flavour than the store-bought ones. Everyone says so.

Raquel beats the eggs and creams the sugar and butter together. She and her husband will eat just a corner of the cake, but there's always somebody stopping by for a meal, you can count on that. When Raquel lived in Whapmagoostui, the community had feasts all the time, and everybody wanted cake at almost every feast, and so Raquel was always baking. Nothing wrong with that.

She pours the batter into the pan, pushes it into the oven, and sets the timer. Her mind goes to her brother who had to move to Montréal for dialysis. Sure would be nice to take him a cake. If she were the one living in Montréal, she'd have a wonderful time. She'd take classes, and beetle around visiting people and window shopping, volunteering with kids and with seniors, do all kinds of city things. But her brother is bored. He doesn't like living in a hotel and longs for the bush. Bored people in cities sometimes seek out the bad undersides just to have something to do. It sure would be good if he could get his dialysis in his home community.

Back when Raquel lived in Moose Factory, the community held regional bingos and raised half the money to buy dialysis machines for the community, and the government matched the money they raised. Then the people with diabetes in Moose Factory who needed dialysis could get it right at home without having to move to the city. Wouldn't it be grand to do something like that in Eeyou Istchee? If they had a bake sale to raise money for dialysis, she'd bake for a year. Nothin' wrong with healthy baking.

Aah, that doc later today will probably disagree. He'll probably just glance at Raquel's shadow, see she's fat, and start in on the judging and the nagging and the giving her hell. You eat too much and that's why you're tired, he'll probably say right off. But Raquel has always been a big girl, has always had a bit of meat on her, even without being a big eater. She worked with a dietician, keeping track of every single mouthful for a whole month, and the dietician said, "I don't know where you're going wrong, Raquel. Except for the occasional bedtime bowl of chips, your diet is pretty much perfect." But the doc probably won't ask if she's worked with a dietician or if she eats carefully. Raquel will probably have to stand up for herself again. Tell him that not everyone who is big eats like a pig. Teach him, like she taught her boys, that every person deserves to be listened to.

Raquel starts cleaning up the kitchen. Dirty dishes in the sink, eggs and leftover butter in the frig, flour and sugar and cocoa in the bottom cupboard, baking powder and flavourings in the top cupboard. She looks in her top cupboard and laughs and laughs. It's so full, she can hardly find space for the tiny bottle of flavouring she took down a few minutes ago. She and her husband might never afford a home of their own, but they could live for a year on what she has crammed into the cupboards. Raquel still lives like she's poor, carefully saving every scrap, always preparing for the rainy day when finances are worse than they are today. Poverty is one of those things you never really forget. If only the doctors understood some of this stuff about their patients, some of the deeper reasons folks do the things they do.

In truth, some of the doctors and nurses are wonderful. They care and really listen. They try to understand the people and not just their diseases. The good docs take the time to explain why a person is sick and how their new medication will fix it and what the person can do to feel better, all without any blaming. And if the med has side effects, the good docs explain that too. You can always tell who the good docs are because their patients really understand what's going on in their own bodies without having to do months of personal research. And without feeling like it's all their fault.

But some of the docs out here get worn down by how busy they are or by all the black flies or something. They just get lost in their judging or their prescribing and don't bother to have a conversation with the people they're supposed to be trying to help. They don't bother to find out what's going on in that person's life that might be making them sick. They don't bother to explain their decisions. Some of Raquel's friends here have felt so bad on meds that they just stopped taking them and didn't bother to tell the doc because he would probably just make them take more pills and they didn't understand why they were taking any in the first place. "Every time I go," her friends say, "It's a different doctor and different pill and no explanation and they're always givin' me hell for something. I'm not a person there. I'm a lab animal to fill with drugs." Some of them stopped going to the doctor altogether. It wasn't worth it.

But Raquel has to go. She's been feeling so tired lately, and the doc ran some tests. She wants to know the results. And she has to stay on top of her diabetes. Sometimes her scrapes and cuts take a bit longer to heal so she has to watch for infection. Good doc or bad doc, she can't skip out on her check-up, ever.

Well, you never know. Maybe today she'll get one of the good ones. Life is hilarious sometimes, so it's best to stay positive and appreciate it.

When Raquel stayed home from school as a teenager to help look after the kids, she also looked after her mom who was sick with diabetes. In those days, the doctors didn't know about proper foot care, or if they did, they never told her mom. Her mom scratched her foot once, who knows on what. It didn't heal and turned septic, and after a while she had to have her foot and lower leg amputated just below the knee.

Later, after the surgery, Raquel asked, "Mom, how do you feel about losing your leg?"

"Well," her mom said, "I look at it this way. That infected foot hurt all the time. It hurt so much that half the time I wanted to die. Now it doesn't hurt. In a few weeks, I'm gonna get a prosthesis and learn to walk on it, so I'll be moving around more than when I had two feet but couldn't walk. I'm alive and not dying of gangrene which is what I was doing when the foot was infected. And I can enjoy my kids and grandkids and even play bingo. I couldn't do any of that when my foot hurt so much it was the only thing I could think about. What I am is grateful."

Raquel listened carefully. That was about the best possible attitude somebody could have about amputation. She and her mom had their tensions, but still there was plenty about her mom to admire.

Diabetes ran through her mom's whole family. Even Raquel's super-skinny aunts had it: they still had their feet, but their sugar levels were all over the place. One thing Raquel learned living with a big family of people with diabetes is that being skinny does not mean you won't get diabetes. Another thing she learned was that exercise helps control diabetes but it won't always prevent it: of Raquel's nine brothers and sisters, all but one developed type 2 diabetes. Even her brother who went all crazy with weightlifting and exercising and living an active life got it in the end.

Sure enough, Raquel walks into the doctor's office and it's a new guy again. He glances at her and says, without even looking at her file, "Raquel, you have to lose weight. You have to eat better."

"That's what the other fella said, and the one before that," she replies, "but I'd appreciate it if you could open that folder and read a little something about the result of my recent thyroid tests."

"Diabetes is serious," he starts.

"I know that," she says. "I've had it for thirty years. If you read my file, you would see that I have taken such good care of myself that I haven't had the troubles that usually come with it. I sure would appreciate hearing about my thyroid, though."

"Thirty years!? Oh! That's, uh, that's different. Here, let me see." He skims her file. "Uh, yes, thirty years. Will you look at that! And they tested your thyroid function. Your thyroid levels are—oh wow, they're too low. Have you felt sluggish lately?"

She just laughs to herself. All that scolding about her eating habits being to blame for low energy, and it turns out she has an energy-sapping thyroid problem. The doctor prescribes thyroid pills and carefully explains what they should do—give her more energy—and what side effects she ought to look out for.

"And you should exercise more," he says.

"Okay, I'll try," she says, and takes the pills from him.

She doesn't tell him that she's not very good at trying to exercise. Sure, a walk makes her feel better for a day or two, and walking with her husband is a nice thing to do in an evening. But they always work so hard just to make ends meet, and do all kinds of community stuff on top of that, so if she has a few minutes at the end of the day, she wants just to sit. *I should go for a walk,* she sometimes thinks, but going for a walk means she won't have any of the sitting-down time she's been looking forward to all day. *It's not worth it,* she thinks then. *I'll stay fat.*

The doc doesn't need to know all that though. He says nothing about his implications that she wasn't taking diabetes seriously or that it had been caused by her girth. But at least he takes the time to explain carefully how her pills work and what she should look for. Best to appreciate the good moments and let the bad ones run off your back.

Well, she better get home. One of her husband's brothers texted—he's bringing his family over for dinner. She has a thawed goose in the frig. She'll rub it down with garlic and other spices and set it to roast. Good thing she baked that cake this morning. In a few hours the house will be full of kids running around and adults trying to outdo each other with dumb jokes.

Makes a good life worth living.

18

The Story of Jack Otter of Waswanipi

IN THE TOWN of Waswanipi, Québec, lives a one-legged man named Jack. If he sees you swimming in the Waswanipi River, he will show you the river bend where he once submerged his legs and a school of hungry river sharks came along and nibbled one right off.

This is not that story.

When Jack Otter was a teenager, his parents lived in the bush. He had to go to school, though, and during the school months he stayed with his aunt in Waswanipi. She was kind and provided a safe home for him in the times he couldn't be with his parents. Still, living on the land was his true way of life and he went out to the bush as often as he could. Like most young Cree in the '80s, Jack could hunt with a gun, but his father had taught him the traditional ways of hunting with bow and arrow or slingshot. An anthropologist came through Eeyou Istchee once and took a photograph of the boy Jack and he published it in a book. In wide-legged stance, Jack is pulling back the band of a slingshot, aiming at some kind of small game.

When Jack was a teenager, he learned that he had diabetes. The nurse said it just meant he should eat a candy if he felt weak and gave him a pamphlet. People with diabetes should eat better, it said, but it didn't explain what "eating better" meant. In fact, it didn't really say anything that made sense to Jack. Obviously, whatever diabetes was, the doctors and nurses weren't taking it seriously so it couldn't be too bad. He wasn't in pain and most of the time he felt fine. It could sometimes be inconvenient—he would run out of energy, or drink jugs of water without quenching his thirst—but it didn't interfere with more important things in life. Like parties on the weekends. Or a quick high now and then. Or the pleasure of a cold beer (or five, or ten) after school with his friends. In his whole life, he would be 18 years old only once. It was important to make the most of it, to have as much fun as he possibly could.

Jack became a conservation officer and, on the side, he studied further to be a game warden. Sometimes at work he suddenly felt much too weak to do the work forestry guys do, and he didn't always remember to carry a piece of candy. When he did remember, the candy worked only a short time; after a half hour or so, he would be right back where he started (asleep in the truck). He didn't know it, but his sudden weakness came from erratic blood sugar levels caused by diabetes. Frustrated and wanting to escape the cycle but not knowing how, Jack began to drink more than before. His sugar levels became even more erratic, and once a month or so he collapsed into a diabetic or hypoglycemic coma and someone would have to take him to the hospital.

The people at the hospital all recognized him. "You must really love it here, Jack," they would joke. "It must be our tasty hospital food. Or comfortable beds. Or maybe it's our cute nurses."

A few days later, with pills or insulin in hand, he'd be back at work again.

All the guys at work knew that forestry jobs involve getting scratched up by branches and insects. No one really complained about it. Jack began to notice that his scratches took weeks to heal but his friends' scratches healed in a few days as usual. Shallow scrapes that barely showed up on Jack's skin began to infect. At the end of the day, when he came home from work, his hands and feet were swollen. He was having a hard time seeing clearly too. Eventually, his vision got so cloudy that he needed laser eye surgery just to be able to do his work. So many health problems. Sure, they all seemed minor, but they were getting to be annoying. If only there were something he could do.

In 2004, Jack was working as a conservation officer in Radisson. He and a friend attended a golf benefit in Val-d'Or and were returning the golf cart to its parking place when they saw something just ahead on the road. Jack's friend swung the driver's wheel to avoid it, and the cart swerved—a little too much. It flipped right over and landed partly on Jack's upside-down leg.

Jack's friend got out and pushed the cart upright again and helped Jack to his feet. But Jack couldn't stand on his leg. It had broken in the accident. His friend took him to the Amos hospital where the doctor set the leg and casted it, gave him something for pain, and Jack went home to Waswanipi to heal.

The leg hurt. It really hurt. Sometimes Jack would wake in the night wanting to vomit, and all day long he felt weak and shaky. It was his first broken bone; probably all healing broken bones felt like this. Still, Jack went to the clinic and asked for a pill to control the nausea and weakness while his leg healed. The doctor eyed him strangely. The pain should have subsided long ago, the doctor said, and nausea and weakness were *not* actually symptoms of broken bones. He reached for his small electric saw, sawed off the cast, and lifted it away.

Jack's leg was obviously infected. The skin was peeling and the area around the break was swollen and shiny and red and purple and green. The infection had filled Jack with toxins and was making him nauseous. Jack didn't know it, but his diabetes was preventing healing; his pancreas was too burned out to create the hormones that help the body heal. The doctor cleaned up the skin, gave Jack antibiotics for the infection. . .

. . . And Jack woke up hundreds of kilometres away in the hospital in Montréal. He had been airlifted there. He remembered none of it. The infection in his broken leg had poisoned his blood so badly that it had even affected his ability to think.

Once Jack was fully awake and alert again, the Montréal doctor told him that, way back on the day of the accident, the doctor in Amos hadn't set the broken leg properly. The bone had been trying to heal for months now, but, because of the improper bone setting and because of his diabetes, it had made no headway at all and was as broken and infected as ever. They re-set the bone then and tried to give the leg another chance to heal. They inserted—right into the flesh—narrow tubes that collected the extra pus and fluids and carried them out of the leg so they couldn't trap toxins inside. They changed the bandages often, always checking the healing flesh very carefully.

Jack hated sitting still. In this Montréal hospital were many other Cree people, so he passed the time by wheeling himself around and visiting them. Some of the older ones didn't speak English or French and were so grateful to have someone there to talk with in their own language. It didn't take long at all for the doctors and nurses to realize what Jack could do, and soon they came for him whenever they had to do a procedure on a Cree person who couldn't speak their languages. Jack wheeled himself into the room and translated for the doctors and the Cree patients. All the while, he visited and joked with the Cree folks in their own language to take their minds off of all of these strange procedures and of the scary place they were in. It felt so good to be useful again. (But what did all the elderly Cree do when no one was there to translate for them? Did they just suffer in fear and silence?)

Eventually, Jack went back home to Waswanipi, where he dutifully stopped by the clinic regularly for check-ups. One day, making his way on crutches around the halls, he hit a patch of wet floor and wiped right out.

CRACK!

A sharp familiar pain shot through his good leg. He had busted his knee. The good one. Of all the dumb luck.

The clinic doctors sent him in an ambulance to the hospital in Chibougamau where a surgeon drilled a plate into the knee to stabilize it so Jack could heal properly. Then came weeks of exercise and rehabilitation, but soon enough the good leg with the busted knee healed.

The other leg, the one broken in the car accident, continued to hurt. One evening, after dinner, Jack began speaking gibberish to his Mom. She looked at him closely, right in the eye—and then called the ambulance. The doctors at the clinic had Jack airlifted to Montréal.

Jack's leg wasn't healing. For six months now, the doctors had tried but the infection continued to eat his leg. In some areas, the flesh was completely gone, and you could see the naked bone that had been broken in the car accident. The pain was unbelievable.

"We're going to have to amputate," the doctor finally said. He was frank and kind all at once. Jack wasn't surprised and nodded his consent.

A week later his lower leg was gone, cut off below the knee.

After that amputation surgery, Jack spent a week in the hospital in the Intensive Care Unit. One day, the machine hooked up to his heart flatlined and sounded the continual beep of someone no longer alive.

Jack's mother was standing there beside the bed when it happened and she slapped him hard: "Stop fooling around, Jack," she shouted and slapped him again. "You better come back or I'm gonna be so mad at you!"

The doctors and nurses went running for the crash cart. Jack knew better than to disobey his mom, though. His heart machine was beating regularly again by the time the cart arrived, and the hospital staff turned right around, taking the crash cart with them.

After Jack had healed further, the doctors fitted him with an artificial leg, a prosthesis. Prostheses, though, are a little bit like cars. You can buy them cheaply made or you can buy them well made. Jack's new leg wasn't the best prosthesis. It rubbed at the stump. It didn't fit properly. It couldn't be locked into place—the whole thing was held in place by a single sheet of rubber at the stump so it would slip off too easily. Sometimes it would drag or slip out of place at a weird angle and people would look at Jack strangely. He would glance down then and see his leg, madly off in all directions. Kind of embarrassing. But it was the prosthesis that the Cree Board of Health paid for. He attached it to his stump as best he could and went back home. Back to work and to beers after work with the boys.

A few weeks later, Jack was having lunch with his mom.

"Mom, when we were in Montréal, we stayed in a hotel room. A really nice expensive room. With a big white bed and white sheets and white curtains that blew in a bit with the breeze and a high white ceiling. People were talking outside the room. Like they were having a party in the hallway. Which hotel was that? How could we afford it?"

She looked at him a little strangely, and said, "Jack, you never stayed in a hotel. You stayed in the hospital and I stayed in a hotel. My hotel wasn't *anything* like that."

"But I remember," he said. "I'm sure of it."

"Boy, you died. That machine went into a flatline. I slapped you around a bit and yelled at you to come back. And it's a good thing you did, or I woulda been *so* mad at you."

That hotel room, it had been real, but it hadn't been in this world.

After Jack had finished all of the physiotherapy and recuperation stuff he was supposed to do, he got ready to head back to work. But just then, his boss called him at home. The company didn't actually *want* Jack back at work as a conservation officer in the field, his boss said. With his new prosthesis, he was able to *do* the work, they could see that, and he had always been a good worker. But they were afraid of being sued if something went wrong for Jack and his artificial leg in the bush. They didn't want the liability. Instead, there was a desk job waiting that they thought would be perfect for him.

Jack didn't want to work at a desk. That was the end of that.

So far Jack had been an optimistic sort of guy. And he had quite a bit of education. He had studied traditional Cree ways on the land, he had studied to be a game warden and a wildlife conservation officer and a firefighter. He could speak three languages. He had options.

But losing a leg and a job in a matter of weeks was a bit much. He let go of his optimism and, for the first time in his life, he began to feel really sorry for himself. He did a whole lot of drinking and a whole lot of sitting around—which led to more diabetic and hypoglycemic comas and hospital stays. He even thought about killing himself and swallowed a bottle of pills. He didn't actually want to die, but his life was turning out so differently from what he had planned and expected. It was confusing. He wanted all this sickness to stop. He wanted comfort and attention. He wanted someone to tell him it would be all right. And it'd sure be nice to have someone tell him what a guy like him was supposed to do now, missing a leg and a job.

The problem was that there *was* no one, really, who could tell him what to do or who could change his situation. As long as he was in a situation he didn't like, and as long as he did nothing about it but drink and sit around, he would continue to be in the situation he didn't like. He had a new son now too. He didn't want his kid to think that his dad had given up.

He would have to figure it out for himself.

Begrudgingly at first, Jack pulled himself together and started to think about other ways he could make a living. He had always wanted to work with kids. He understood them. He had taken a course in suicide prevention—funny for a guy who had swallowed a bottle of pills—and he knew some Cree kids were in trouble. Maybe he had something to offer.

But that leg, the bad leg that had already been amputated, was bothering him again. The prosthesis rubbed badly against the stump. Sometimes the skin rubbed right off and then it got infected and he would have to go to Montréal for infection control and it was all so familiar.

Wouldn't you know—Jack was in the hospital being treated for infection in the stump, and again they had the drains carrying fluid out of the flesh, and again they were washing the area with antibiotics and applying treatments, and again the treatments weren't working and the flesh was being eaten away, and again the doctor took a look. And said they were going to have to amputate. The same leg, up higher, above the knee. Again.

Jack swore in Cree. He really wanted to swear in English and French too, but he didn't want the doctors and nurses there to know he was swearing. So he just swore some more in Cree and the others in the room heard some words they had probably never heard before.

A few days after that, he went into surgery and woke up after. His leg stump now ended in the middle of his thigh bone.

Last time, Jack had been eaten up with anger and self-pity and it hadn't helped at all. If he didn't want to go through the whole stupid situation a third time, he was going to have to help himself. The prosthesis provided by the Cree Board of Health was not the prosthesis that Jack needed, he knew that now. His flesh infected so easily that he needed a much more expensive prosthesis, one that fit securely and could be locked into position and wouldn't rub off his skin. One that cost ten thousand dollars more than the prosthesis CBH provided. Jack would have to pay the difference himself.

Ten thousand dollars was a whole lot more money than Jack had. Either he had to come up with it or he had to get ready for the whole infection-amputation cycle to begin again. On crutches, Jack went to the bank, got a loan, and bought himself the expensive artificial leg. The situation was annoying—but at least he had been able to do something about it. After the new leg had been properly fitted, he went home, rested both legs on the coffee table and had a few beers to unwind.

Diabetic and hypoglycemic comas, and the inevitable hospital stays that came with them, were still a big part of Jack's life. Sometimes, as he injected himself with insulin, he wondered if his drinking had something to do with them, but surely, if that were the case, a doctor or nurse would have mentioned it somewhere along the way.

"You're going to need dialysis soon," a nurse said one day. "It's pretty clear that your kidneys are giving out. Will you be moving to Montréal, then, do you think?"

Jack smiled politely but didn't answer. His kidneys? He knew people on dialysis. Their lives were much more restricted than he wanted ever to be. He needed to be able to go to the bush. He needed to be able to hunt and fish. He needed to be able to move around Eeyou Istchee. Dialysis simply was not an option.

As soon as he was able, Jack began looking online for options other than dialysis. He found one—and it was every bit as drastic as amputation. He could have his kidney cut out and replaced with a transplanted kidney. He could also, at the same time, have his burnt-out pancreas replaced with a transplanted one. The doctors had always told him that there was no cure for diabetes. Once diabetic, always diabetic. But if he got a new pancreas, one not burnt out by diabetes, there was a chance that he might truly be cured.

At his next check-up in Montréal, Jack asked the doctor about transplanted organs.

"Oh Jack. I don't think you'd be a good candidate for that," the doctor said. "That's more a solution for—other people. But you could try dialysis. It's not so bad, you know. Lots of folks around here do it."

Jack smiled politely—then drove across town to the transplant clinic, where he asked question after question. Before transplant surgeons would even consider him for a transplant, the people at the clinic said, Jack would have to have his diabetes under better control and be regularly eating a healthy diet. Even harder, he would have to stop drinking altogether. If he managed to do those two things, then he might be eligible. If he was eligible, he'd be put on a list. After that, he would have to wait and see if anyone with healthy matching tissues died and donated her or his organs to people who needed them. If Jack got the organs, he would have to take special pills and he'd have to exercise and eat healthy and never drink alcohol and never get high for the rest of his life. It would be a big big deal and maybe in the end there would be no organs for him. But he could try. And he was getting pretty tired of comas and hangovers anyways. They had lost their appeal a long time ago.

Jack quit drinking and he quit doing drugs. It was not easy at all. It was probably the hardest thing he had ever done. He attended no Alcoholics Anonymous nor Narcotics Anonymous group—Waswanipi had no such groups back then—and he had no support group. In fact, he had to stop hanging out with some of his closest friends for a while because, even though they were good people, when he was with them he wanted to drink. What he had was the knowledge that if he quit drinking and quit drugs, he stood a chance at a good life without dialysis; if he didn't quit, he had no chance at all. And he had the bush. Every time he wanted to drink, he went fishing, or for a drive, or out on the land. For a long time, it seemed that Jack spent most of his time fishing, driving, or out in the bush. That part wasn't so bad. The bush had always been his favourite place to be.

Jack began to speak with the new nutritionist who worked at the Waswanipi clinic. She explained to him what a healthy diet actually was and how diabetes works in the body, and she taught him ways to manage his diabetes with food. There were foods that made it worse (breads, sugars, beer, pastas) and foods that helped (traditional meats, vegetables). In fact, he learned, there were quite a few things he could have done a long time ago to help manage the disease. He just hadn't known about them. Or if he had known, he hadn't taken them seriously. Five months after his last drink and after starting to eat differently, he drove himself back down to the transplant clinic in Montréal.

They looked him over carefully and asked him questions. Organ transplant is one of the most extreme surgeries that can be done so they had to be sure that his heart was strong enough to survive the surgery. And there are more people who need organs than who ever receive them so they had to be sure that Jack would respect the new organs. If he went back to a life of drinking and of eating in unhealthy ways, he would burn out the organs very quickly. And anyone who has had a transplant has to take pills to convince the immune system to accept the new organs. Those pills can't be forgotten even once. Their list of questions and tests was long and intense. But, by the time Jack left the clinic, he was on a list for new organs. If someone with healthy organs and matching tissues died, he could receive their organs.

In the meantime, the doctors put him on temporary dialysis. His own kidneys could no longer flush out all the toxins they were supposed to flush out, but his blood had to be free of toxins if he was to live through such a rigorous surgery. For two months, he went into the Montréal dialysis clinic three times a week and sat there for four hours as the big dialysis machine cleaned his blood. Again, he met many Cree people there who needed someone to talk to and Jack was happy to oblige.

One day, he heard that someone had died too soon and organs had become available for him. But for some reason Jack had a fever that day and his surgery had to be cancelled. The organs went to someone else on the list. Not too long after that, Jack was about to catch a plane to Waswanipi for a visit when someone else died too soon. Jack stayed in Montréal and, on that day in 2012, he received a new kidney and a new pancreas.

Jack is the one person in this book who once had diabetes but no longer does. Because he has a new pancreas, and because his body accepts the insulin it creates, he is actually cured of the disease. His new pancreas works beautifully, and his new kidney feels fine. But transplanted organs have to be handled very carefully. Even though he no longer has diabetes, he is more vigilant about health than he ever was before. He avoids fast food, he cooks his own meals (mostly meat and vegetables with a little bit of pasta or potatoes), and he doesn't drink or do drugs even a little bit. Since the bush is where he has always felt healthiest, he spends as much time on the land as he can. He teaches his son the traditional ways of the land so that his son knows that even a robot leg and transplanted organs can't stop you from living on the land if it's what you want to do. He hunts and brings home moose and other game, and he cooks it up. He exercises when he can. His lower back often aches from the extra work it has to do with an artificial leg and his flesh-and-blood foot sometimes gets swollen from all the exercise, but exercise is what has to happen if he wants to stay healthy, and so Jack does it. When he's stressed out about life in general, he talks with an elder, and when he's stressed out about work, he talks to a psychologist so the stress doesn't bottle up inside.

Sometimes he thinks about bullshit. He heard piles of it over the years. Maybe if someone had been direct with him when he was younger, his diabetes would not have become so severe and he might still have his original leg and kidney and pancreas. Sometimes he still runs into bullshit. A counsellor told him not long ago that he had to accept that his time in the bush was over, that hunting was not something a one-legged man should do. Jack smiled politely— then left the clinic to go hunting. The way to deal with bullshit is to help yourself.

Not long ago, someone asked him if he felt like his new organs had given him a second chance. He thought about it for a while.

"Not a second chance, exactly," he said. "I feel like the Lord came through. But a little too late."

He's not angry at the doctors who made so many mistakes, and he doesn't want to sue anyone for malpractice. He told a friend once that, if he had sued back when his leg had to be amputated because of a doctor's mistake, he would just have had more money, which he would have spent on more drinking and partying, which would have led to even more health problems. Nor is he angry at his bosses who didn't want the liability of having him working in forestry. He's not even angry at the people who provided a cheap prosthesis that only irritated his leg further and led to a second amputation. What he wants is to move on, to continue to live the good life he has, to contribute in meaningful ways.

He works as a counsellor and suicide prevention officer with the youth of Waswanipi, is on the Board of Directors for First Nations and Inuit of Québec and Labrador, and is the co-president of Suicide Prevention in the region. He also works with the Cree Board of Health to protect the livelihoods of people with disabilities, he and his wife foster kids and provide a safe home for them when they can't be with their parents, and he is on call with Youth Protection.

The youth he works with have heard piles of bullshit too. So he tells them direct, straight off the bat, "Look, this is what you gotta do. If you don't do it, this is what will happen." He tells them to look after themselves, or to stop drinking, or to eat healthier, or to stop fighting, or to do whatever they can do to improve their situation. He tells them the truth, all of it, including how they can help themselves, including that it's up to them to make their own lives better. When he says that, they look at his robot leg and believe him.

He still thinks of all the Cree who suffer alone in the hospitals. Eventually, after his son is grown and has learned about life on the land, Jack and his wife might move to Montréal where he might work as a counsellor and translator in the hospitals. For now, this is where he should be.

19

The Story of Lillian Martinhunter of Chisasibi

LILLIAN Martinhunter loved kids. They would make all kinds of mess and noise, and she was always cleaning up after them or chasing them down from one thing or another or bracing for another yell. Those things didn't bother her at all. When there weren't enough kids around, the world was too quiet for Lillian.

She and her husband had six kids. The youngest was still a toddler, not yet in school, when Lillian said to her husband, "I think I want to adopt a child. Maybe a little girl. Or a little boy."

"A *seventh* kid!? Who will look after it?" her husband said. "We're both working."

But after another 15 years or so, after all six of their kids were grown and her husband retired, the house seemed too quiet for both of them. There was a baby girl from Nunavut, a relative of Lillian's husband, who needed a home. It didn't take long at all for Lillian and her husband to adopt her.

Every night, Lillian's husband would tuck their new daughter into bed. He had severe rheumatoid arthritis and couldn't lift her, but he could cook her dinner and give her a bath at night and read her stories and sing to help her fall asleep. Until she was two years old, when he died of a heart attack, he took care of her. After he passed away, Lillian would come home from her work with Youth Protection to a house even emptier than it had been before. She was more grateful than ever for her daughter's company, for the day she heard about a little Inuk girl who needed a home.

After a few years, the little girl began to ask questions: "Where did I come from?"

"You came from Nunavut, in the North. The day I got the call, I was ready to pick you up."

"Why did you take me from my mom?" she asked. And "Why did my mom let me go?"

"We really needed another daughter," Lillian said. "And your mother was very sick. She was worried that she would get sicker and maybe even die and if that happened you wouldn't have a mother at all. We came to get you so that you would have a mother and a father and so that we would have another daughter."

Around that time, Lillian packed a suitcase for both of them and they flew up north to the town her daughter was from. It was the first time the girl was back where she had been born. When they got off the plane, the airport was full of people. Lillian had never seen so many people there before. It seemed like every family in town was in that airport, all wanting to see the Inuk girl from their town and her Cree mother.

After that, Lillian took her daughter north about once a year so that she knew where she was from. They would visit for a few days.

Lillian thought that maybe her daughter would grow up to be a veterinarian, or to build an animal shelter. Her daughter loved animals, especially the Chisasibi dogs. She didn't like to see them suffer, she wished they were all fed and had enough water and exercise and were well looked after. She wanted to make life better for every one of them.

Lillian used to eat baskets of french fries with ketchup. And white bread with strawberry jam. And doughnuts. And bannock.

She especially loved big meals with chicken or pork and with mashed potatoes that were slathered in butter. In 2006, when her daughter was four years old, Lillian was working on her Bachelor of Arts in Social Work at the University of Québec. She and some other students and her colleagues were researching a project in English Literature. They had spread books across the table and Lillian sat at the computer typing in notes of everything they said. She reached for her glass of juice, emptied it quickly, and went back to typing.

"Lillian, that's your fourth glass of apple juice."

"Yeah, I'm thirsty. Uh, what did that book say again?" She sat, poised over the computer.

"And before, you went through a litre of juice."

"Yeah, I was thirsty. My mouth is kind of dry."

"And yesterday you drank that whole four-litre jug of water."

"Yeah, I was thirsty."

"Don't drink anything for an hour now, okay? I'm going to test your blood sugar then."

"Sure, whatever." And they went back to work.

An hour later, her colleague pricked Lillian's finger with a little lancet, smeared some blood on a test strip, and slid the test strip into a glucometer she had.

Lillian's blood sugar level was over 15.

"Lillian, this is serious. You have to stop drinking juice right now. Drink water. And tomorrow you have to go to the doctor and tell him you have very high blood sugar and you're thirsty all the time."

The next day, the doctor said that anyone with a blood sugar level of 15 had diabetes. Lillian had diabetes.

That was quick, Lillian thought. Her mother had had diabetes. She had lived a long life. And then, in her late '70s, she had gall bladder surgery and, because of her diabetes, it hadn't healed properly. One thing led to another until she passed away. Two of

Lillian's brothers had diabetes too. But Lillian hadn't thought it would happen to her. Or if it did, certainly not so soon: she exercised all the time. She was the only adult in her house, and she shovelled the snow and chopped the wood and did whatever needed to be done. For the days that yard work and household chores weren't enough, she had a treadmill in her basement. Diabetes was the last thing she expected would happen to her.

Well. Lillian thought back to her mom. *Diabetes is serious. Now things will have to change.* She made an appointment to see a dietician and get the details. And that was the end of Lillian's french fries and doughnuts and white bread with strawberry jam. It was the end of drinking juice and the end of dessert. Except for some small treats from time to time, she cut sugars and starchy foods right out of her diet.

Over the next years, Lillian switched away from big meals altogether. She stopped eating until she was full and instead ate only until she was satisfied. But she ate more often: usually six little meals a day. In each meal, she had a bit of fish or moose or caribou or game bird like partridge or ptarmigan along with something else, maybe a vegetable. Before, Lillian hadn't noticed feeling sick. But now, with all the traditional meats, regular small meals, and never eating until she was full, her blood sugar levelled right off. She felt so much better that the change wasn't hard to make at all.

The thing about having all those kids—they had had kids of their own, Lillian's grandkids. And some of those grandkids loved to hunt. When they heard their grandma had diabetes, they filled her freezer with hunted game and fish. Lillian began to cook traditional food as often as she could.

Lillian's daughter liked the taste of the hunted game—but she felt so sorry for the animals.

"Do we really have to eat caribou, Mom?" she said, as Lillian's grandson hefted a hind quarter into the freezer. "They're so beautiful and they have to migrate so far. After all that walking and running, they die and end up on our plate. Couldn't we take this caribou outside for the dogs and leave all the other caribou alive?"

One day, Lillian thought, *that girl is going to be a vegetarian.*

Sometimes Lillian would crave chocolate—and so she'd have some. Sometimes she would eat too much bread—and when she did that, she would cut out a different starchy food later on, like bannock or dumplings. Sometimes, she couldn't stop thinking about apple juice—and then she would eat some unsweetened applesauce instead.

Lillian was one of the lucky ones. She was controlling her diabetes mostly through diet and the exercises she had always done. If her blood sugar climbed a bit too high for one reason or another, she exercised and it came right down. She took some insulin at night before she went to bed, just in case, but, for Lillian, all those other changes were not hard to make.

In 2010, a mammogram trailer came to Chisasibi. All women, the doctors said, should go to the trailer and have their breasts scanned for tumours. Between her shifts with Youth Protection, Lillian went over to the trailer for the routine test. She wasn't sick, it would be fine.

It wasn't fine. She had breast cancer. A few weeks later, Lillian flew to Montréal where she checked into a hospital and the surgeons did a lumpectomy and cut a cancerous tumour out from her breast.

Soon after Lillian had recovered from her surgery, the doctors began to give her chemotherapy. Once a week, they pumped a special medication into her veins, a medication that was actually poison. The poison was supposed to kill off any remaining cancer cells. It also made her want to throw up.

After her second treatment, Lillian was taking a shower—but the shower wasn't draining properly and she was standing in water.

She looked down at the drain. It was completely clogged by her beautiful thick straight hair which was falling out in big clumps. A few days later, Lillian was completely bald. She rummaged through her closet and pulled out her warmest hat to cover her cold head.

As soon as the chemotherapy was done, and her hair began to grow in again, curly this time, the doctors began to give her radiation treatments. They aimed a radioactive beam at her breast, just in case a few tiny cells had missed the knife and also survived the chemotherapy poison. Of all the things Lillian went through with breast cancer, the surgery and the chemotherapy and the nausea and the baldness and everything, the radiation was the worst part. It actually burnt her breast.

Lillian was never one to complain. She saw women in the radiation unit who had lost their breasts altogether, and she was much better off than they were. But through the months of dealing with cancer, she had thought back many times to her mother who had died of diabetes-related complications from surgery. Chemotherapy, especially, drove up Lillian's blood sugar, and she worried.

In the end, it was okay. They got rid of all the cancer, every bit of it, she had no diabetes complications from the surgery, and she healed just fine.

These days, Lillian has 7 children, 30 grandchildren and 5 great-grandchildren. She likes it best when they're all there, at her house. They make all kinds of mess and noise, and she's forever cleaning up after them or chasing them down from one thing or another or bracing for yet another yell. That's just fine with her.

After they leave and it's just Lillian and her teenage daughter, the girl says to her, "The house is too quiet now, Mom. Don't you think we should bring in some dogs, just to make some noise?"

Stories We Heard Along the Way: Travels

One of the food organizers for a health conference took health seriously, so he had arranged for all the conference food to be healthy food. No junk food, no poutine, and no pop. The conference lasted a few days, and after it was finished, the organizer was escorted to the plane—the people who remained behind wanted to make sure he left so that they could go back to their poutine. But then the plane didn't arrive because of bad weather and the organizer walked back to town, back to the conference venue. When he stepped again into the building, the people looked up from their junk food and poutine and pop and asked, "What are you doing here? We just got rid of you!"

•

A Cree health worker was in Chisasibi, on her way up to Whapmagoostui. In the Chisasibi airport, a woman asked her if she was flying north, and then asked her to take along a three-month-old baby boy to visit his grandmother in Whapmagoostui. The health worker agreed and took the baby on the flight. She didn't know the name of the boy, the names of his mom and grandmother, the address of the home to which he was going or from where he had come, nor anything about the boy at all. Once the plane arrived in Whapmagoostui, another woman approached her. "There's my grandson," she said. "Thank you for bringing him." Later, when telling the story, the health worker said she had known it would all work out because the mother spoke Cree. Then she laughed, "Only in the Cree nation. Only in the Cree nation."

•

Many years ago, before the time of satellite phones and cell towers, a missionary bush pilot was approached by a local Cree man who had Sight. "Take your plane," the man said, pointing to a map, "and fly here. I had a vision. There's a man who's been injured and needs help." He gave the missionary all the important details he would need to find the man and bring him back safely. With nothing but the man's vision to go on, the missionary was reluctant to go: fuel was expensive, and what if he flew all the way there only to find nothing but trees and wildlife? The man persisted, however, and finally the missionary relented, just to keep the peace. He got up in his plane, landed on the assigned lake, and found the man who needed help, exactly as had been described to him. After that, whenever a Cree person said he or she had Sight, the missionary didn't question it. He also didn't question the motive: traditionally, if someone has Sight and uses it for personal gain, she or he loses it.

•

Overheard in Eastmain airport:
Airport worker: I need to see your identification.
Traveller: But—we grew up together. We live on the same street. We see each other every day. You know me!
Airport worker: Yup. I know you. I need to see your identification.

•

Also overheard in Eastmain airport:
Airport worker: We have to weigh your luggage. Bring it to the scale.
Traveller: I'm sitting now. You're closer, you do it. It's the red bag.

20

The Story of Caroline Neeposh of Chisasibi

WHEN you really have the taste for rabbit, you make it like this: Skin the rabbit. Set aside the fur and skin—you can use it later to edge leather mitts but you don't need it now. With a strong knife or cleaver, chop the rabbit into pieces, drop the pieces into a pot, and add enough water to cover it. With the lid on, bring the pot to a rolling boil, and then turn the burner down. Simmer that rabbit slowly, so that the juices run out into the water and the slow boil softens the flesh. Add some salt and pepper, not much. Just let that tender meat be. After it has simmered for an hour or two, pour the liquid into another pot, stir in some flour to thicken the gravy and heat it, stirring constantly, until the gravy boils. Now drop dollops of dumpling dough into the boiling gravy. Cover the pot and don't lift the lid for about 15 minutes, so the dumplings can steam. Pour it all—gravy, dumplings, rabbit—into a big bowl and serve it like that. You need patience to be a good cook. Patience and an understanding of the different meats go further than any seasonings.

Caroline had patience, plenty of patience. That's why she was such a good cook.

The La Tuque Residential School, where Caroline was sent when she was young, had a Yardstick Policy. If any student talked back or broke one of the bewildering rules, all the students would be called to the dining room. They would be lined up against a long table and made to bend over it, chests to the tabletop. Then the priest would fetch his yardstick, lift his arm high, and crack the stick down on each child's backside, one by one. It was a big school in those days, with many rules and many kids to break them: Caroline and her friends spent plenty of time bent over dining room tables, clenching against the yardstick. There wasn't anything they could do about it but wait for things to change.

And then that priest got sent away and things at La Tuque got better for everyone.

Years passed. Caroline finished her schooling, married, and moved away from her home in Mistissini to Chisasibi to live with her new husband. They lived in a three-bedroom house and had some good times. Like when they sat down together to dinner. She would set a freshly roasted goose on the table and they would look at the platter together for a minute, the dark steaming bird circled by rice or dumplings. Then they'd both reach in and rip off a drumstick. As she ate, she would watch him—when his mouth was full of goose, his eyes closed in pleasure. What a wonderful meal, what a very fine cook she was, he would say across the table. After dinner they'd relax, just the two of them, over a quiet drink. It was something to do.

The bad times came about half an hour later, when she was still nursing her first drink, sipping it slowly, and he was on his third. Or fourth. Then sometimes he would hit her. It was the Yardstick Policy all over again—why had he hit her? What rule had she broken? She would have to wait. Things would change eventually.

After a couple of years like this, Caroline learned she was going to have a baby and that even slow drinking could hurt the baby. So she stopped. It wasn't hard. She hadn't been drinking much anyways. She had a healthy baby boy, and then, not long after, another one. Sometimes her husband still got angry—and by the time the third boy came along, she was drinking a little bit again. Not a lot; she never got really drunk; it was something to do to pass the long evenings. And to take her mind off things.

One day, Caroline had to pay someone a visit. Her kids were sleeping. She laid out clothes for each boy, called in the babysitter, and told her which boy should go into which clothes. Then she went out.

An hour later she came back. The babysitter and her boyfriend were passed out drunk on the sofa—and the kids were gone. Their clothes were still nicely laid out in their rooms where Caroline had left them. There was no note, no way to know where the kids were, if they had run out to play, or if someone had taken them.

Caroline was sick with worry but she wasn't sure what to do. She waited. When her husband came home, she told him and he called Social Services. Maybe they would know something about the kids.

It turned out that Caroline's sons, still in their pajamas, had been taken by Social Services. A neighbour had called and said the parents were drinking. A hard month later, Caroline had her kids back.

Not long after that, it happened again and nearly the same way. She left the kids with someone to look after them; she and her husband had business an hour away in Radisson. When they came back, the kids were gone, taken into foster care again, this time all the way down to Wemindji. Someone had called Social Services and said she was drinking.

Another month and Caroline had her kids back again. But this time they told her how unhappy they had been in the foster homes hundreds of kilometres away. One of her sons crawled into her lap and said he had gotten into trouble for fighting. Caroline held him and listened to him and didn't say anything. In all the years he had lived with her, he hadn't been in a single fight.

Caroline had never been so sad. Why was this happening? Why didn't Social Services try to take the kids when she was there? When she could explain that she was a slow drinker, never really drunk. If she waited, would things get better?

Now she was under more stress than ever.

Now, she really started drinking.

In the next few years, Caroline gave birth to two more boys, and she went into alcohol addiction recovery twice. At the second recovery centre, in New Brunswick, she decided she was done with drinking. It had taken the edge off, but her life wasn't getting better, and she wasn't forgetting any of the stuff she wanted to forget.

On weekends in rehab, Caroline worked in the kitchen. Everyone there loved her cooking. Staff and recovering addicts stopped her in the hallways and asked when her next shift was—they were looking forward to her food. When her rehabilitation program ended, the recovery centre administration asked her to please stay in New Brunswick. Stay and be their cook. But Caroline had to rush home, back to Chisasibi. Christmas was coming and she wanted to be with her kids.

Back home, she found work as a cleaner in a restaurant. She was sober now—and that meant she had more money in her wallet, she felt healthier without the alcohol in her system, and Social Services wouldn't have reason to take her kids. Her days at work were long, and then she came home and cooked for the kids, and also tried to stay out of the way of her husband when he had one of those moods. She was a little tired. And sometimes she was so sad. But everyone got tired or sad, didn't they? She would just keep at it until something changed.

Over the next ten years, as Caroline kept at it, kept working, first as a cleaner and then as a dishwasher, she collapsed twice. Twice she was med-evaced to Montréal. Twice the diagnosis was the same: exhaustion and depression. Twice she stayed in the hospital for several months, gradually healing, gradually getting stronger. She felt safe there, with others looking after her. Safe enough even to admit that she was not only sad—but very very angry. Sometimes, she was so angry that the doctor tied down her wrists to keep her from hurting herself. And then, both times, when she felt better again, she returned home to Chisasibi.

In 2003, Caroline was cleaning her house. She swept a room, picked up a stuffed toy, and sat down for a minute. She got up again, swept the next room, and put away the clothes the kids had dropped on the floor and sat for a minute. For four years, she had worked only part-time because she didn't want to get over-tired again and be sent to Montréal. But even so, she was tired now, more tired than usual. Her mouth opened in a huge yawn. Something wasn't quite right. Well, it was time she had a doctor's check-up anyways.

At the clinic, they did all the usual tests. The good news was that Caroline didn't have to be med-evaced. The bad news was that she had diabetes. Other than feeling tired, she had noticed no diabetes symptoms. She had not felt sick at all.

Caroline listened to the nurse and yawned. She wasn't really surprised. Diabetes ran in her family. Long ago, a doctor had said that, sometimes, stress or alcohol could increase your chances of diabetes. She had had quite a bit of both in her life.

The nurse was still talking. Now, she said, Caroline would have to start taking insulin—and she should also change her diet, reduce the stress in her life, and exercise every day. Caroline listened and didn't say anything. She could take the medication and change her diet. That much she could manage. But first, she needed a nap.

Over the next days, Caroline learned the insulin ritual. Push a syringe into an insulin bottle, pull back the plunger to suck up the fluid, roll up her shirt, slide the needle into her stomach flesh, and push down the plunger to ease the medication into her body. Later, the doctor added pills too. When she was very careful, and took the pills and injections at exactly the right time, she felt better right away. As if she had been feeling poorly for years without even knowing it.

She changed her cooking too. Less flour and sugar. No more dessert. No packaged foods (they made her feel terrible). More traditional foods. She told her sons she had diabetes. They didn't say anything. They just took their guns and went out to their trap-lines more often. Now her kitchen filled with the smells of partridge and rabbit and caribou every week—and no one complained about that.

Unfortunately, her husband still lost his temper sometimes. When that happened, she would say to him, "Fine. Just hit me already. Get it over with." And then he did.

But something in Caroline had changed. She was getting used to taking medication that made her feel better, getting used to cooking the foods her body needed and staying away from those that made her sick. She was getting used to looking after herself. In 2009, she woke her husband when he was sleeping. He lost his temper and said some of the most awful things she had ever heard, then stormed out of the bedroom. She lay back on the bed for a while, and looked up at the ceiling, thinking. She had diabetes now. She couldn't wait for things to get better. She had to do something about the stress.

Caroline got up from the bed. She went to the closet and took down a big bag. She packed her medication, some clothes for herself and for her youngest son. The two of them drove to the air-port, flew down to Montréal, and went to the women's shelter. The people at the shelter welcomed them and gave them a comfortable room and good meals. And when they heard her story, they told her to go to the police and press charges against her husband. They showed her where the police station was. At the station, the people listened to her, and, after all those years, Caroline's husband went to court and had to answer for the things he had done to her. And Caroline, run down from the stress and upheaval of it all, had to check into the hospital for several months a third time, again with exhaustion and depression.

After all that was finished, and she had recovered and was back at home, alone with her husband again, he told her something she had not heard before. He was so angry, so very angry, because of the terrible things done to him when he was a small boy in residential school. And he apologized to her. It didn't fix the things he had done but now she understood why he had done them. She had waited a very long time for that.

Caroline and her husband live together in Chisasibi with three of their five kids. They have been married for 33 years and their kids are all grown. Her husband no longer hits her, nor shouts at her, nor drinks. They have no liquor in their house. He's good company now and it's nice to have him around. She looks forward to spending more days with him. Her blood sugar is levelling out and she takes less insulin now than she once did. The family eats as much traditional food as they can—her roasted goose and stewed rabbit are the favourites—and often, when she's cooking, one of her sons will come through the kitchen and give her a peck on the cheek.

Caroline should exercise more, the doctor says. Maybe she will, some day.

21

The Story of Jonathan Linton of Mistissini

JONATHAN stepped out of the truck, sidled up to a bush, unzipped his jeans, and peed into the October snow. He zipped up, climbed back into the truck, and his dad slid it into gear again. They drove slowly, looking out carefully for tracks or disturbed foliage, any hint that a porcupine or partridge had passed by. Moose would be nice. Jonathan still hadn't shot a moose. He twisted the cap off his water bottle and sucked back a mouthful. Strange how dry his mouth was. This morning's kill, a pair of geese, sat in the back of the truck. They inched forward again.

Except—Jonathan had to pee. Again. His dad stopped the truck. This was ridiculous.

He'd peed *eight* times in the last hour. How could one human body even make that much pee? What was the point in doing up his fly if he was just gonna have to pee again? And his mouth. He could write a letter on his tongue, it was so dry. *Focus,* he told himself. Jonathan had done quite a bit of hunting. Shot his first partridge when he was six. Now, he knew, was the time to concentrate—but he felt *awful*.

Dry mouth. Frequent urination. He'd seen those words somewhere on a list. No, on a poster about—diabetes? Jonathan was young and fit and healthy. A 15-year-old hunter and high school student and enforcer on the Mistissini Bears hockey team. It couldn't be diabetes.

Could it?

A few days later, Jonathan sat at the kitchen table and read the instructions on a diabetes test kit. He inserted a test strip into the glucometer device, unwrapped the lancet in the kit, and pricked his finger. He carefully smeared some blood onto the test strip. A blood sugar level below 6 was normal, he knew, between 6 and 7 was pre-diabetes, a warning sign that diabetes was just around the corner, and anything over 7 was diabetes.

He looked at the glucometer. It said his blood sugar level was 32.2. That *couldn't* be right. A reading of over 30 meant he had to be hospitalized immediately because he could slip into a coma. He took the test again. 32.1. And again and again and again. All the numbers were about the same. No question, Jonathan had diabetes.

He got up from his chair, went to the clinic, where they injected him with insulin. An hour later, he felt better.

But now he had a problem: his blood sugar levels meant that he should be in the Chibougamau hospital where the doctors and nurses could watch him. His mother was a Community Health Representative (CHR), and she would make him go, he was sure— and that would ruin his weekend plans. He and some friends from football camp were going to Montréal to watch the Montréal Alouettes game and then all meet with them. Jonathan would have supper with the quarterback and be in a commercial with him. It was a big deal and he didn't want to miss it.

Methodically, purposefully, he began to persuade his mom to let him go on the trip. He could take needles and insulin, he rea-soned. He would follow the injection rules perfectly. He would text her throughout the weekend and keep her updated. She didn't need to be afraid for him, he'd be careful, he'd be okay. Besides, if anything went wrong, Montréal had hospitals. In the end, she came around.

He still had another problem, though: he needed to keep the diabetes secret. He packed the insulin carefully, tucking it first inside a sock and then rolling the socks into underwear, stuffing it all way down in his bag, where no one would see it. All weekend long, he faithfully texted his mom for advice. Did toast affect blood sugar? (Yes) Did chewing gum affect blood sugar? (No) But he told no one about the diabetes, not his friends, not the trip organizers, and certainly not the Alouettes quarterback. And he didn't take the insulin nearly as often as he should have. *It's hard to inject*, he said to himself. *Insulin has to go into fat. I'm an athlete. Lots of muscle, not a lot of fat.* But in truth, he wasn't taking enough insulin because he didn't want to be seen with insulin.

The football trip was fine and Jonathan didn't get sick, but when he came home, he headed straight for the bedroom and flipped on the TV. And stayed there for days. He didn't go to school. He didn't go to his hockey practices. He didn't go to his hockey games. He didn't see a diabetes specialist.

After a week, his bedroom began to smell a bit ripe.

After two weeks, his dad said, "Look. Television doesn't actually make diabetes go away. Go to school. You can still do everything you did before, you can still be whatever you want to be, unless you don't finish high school. Diabetes isn't the end of the world."

The next day, Jonathan was back in school and playing hockey again. The school principal asked where he'd been. "I went to the clinic and then I stayed home," he said, and looked away. No way was he saying *anything* about diabetes.

He went to a diabetes specialist that week too. She said that some people can eventually control diabetes by changing their diet and increasing exercise, but for now Jonathan would have to take either pills or insulin, and most people started with pills. His body needed more insulin, insulin is made in the pancreas, and pills would make the pancreas work harder. Eventually it would burn out, she said, and pancreas burnout is when people usually start injecting insulin with needles.

"Wouldn't it make more sense," Jonathan asked, "if I skipped pills and just injected insulin? I'd be giving my pancreas a break."

"Yes," she said, "but do you know how many needles that will be?"

Jonathan was used to flying pucks, body checks, concussions, broken limbs, and bruises. He was the enforcer on his hockey team, the goon. His job was to do the hitting on the ice, and even to try to aggravate players on the other team and make them screw up. A bunch of little needles every day were not a big deal. As long as no one saw them.

Jonathan began to eat more carefully—fewer carbohydrates, less junk food, less frequent snacking—and took his insulin religiously, one shot every time he ate and another before bed. He worked out even more than he had before. After a few months, he needed about half as much insulin and another month later, half of that. Soon he wasn't using insulin or any diabetes medication at all. He had made important progress: he had brought severe diabetes under control. But he still didn't tell anyone that he had the disease.

It has to be secret, he said to himself as he bench-pressed the barbell. *It's dangerous to tell people,* he thought, hoisting his chin over the chin-up bar. Anybody at school who was a little bit different was bullied regularly. Like that girl who got harassed and called a slut just because she wore a bit of eye makeup. The toughest guy in school was already beating Jonathan up for being half-Cree, half-white. *If they find out I'm diabetic too, I'll never make it home,* he thought, straining against the plates on the leg machine.

At school one day, Jonathan stood at the sink in the bathroom. The door swung open and the toughest guy in school walked in and came at Jonathan as he had so many times before. "White boy" he jeered, and kneed him in the stomach.

Jonathan didn't think about how frustrated he was with the tough guy, nor about his diabetes secret, nor about how much stronger all the extra workouts had made him. He just wound up and landed one solid punch to the forehead. The guy buckled and hit the ground. He lay there on his back for a while, then got up and never bothered Jonathan again. Soon after that, the school brought in an anti-bullying program. Things were beginning to change. Jonathan began to think about letting his secret out.

Tentatively, hesitantly, Jonathan mentioned to one of his friends that he had diabetes. "Huh," his friend said—and began avoiding him, as if he had something contagious instead of diabetes. Some things, like being treated badly in high school if you were different, would probably never change. For Jonathan, secrecy was still the way to go.

The year Jonathan turned 16, he killed a bear. 24 feet away, 7 mm with a scope. Like the elders taught, he was careful to make full eye contact with the bear before shooting. The diabetes was still a secret.

The year Jonathan turned 17, a Junior AAA hockey team wanted him to be their enforcer. It didn't work out, and he could try again next year, but it was nice to be asked. That year, he had to start taking insulin again too. And the diabetes was still a secret.

Around that time, the Cree Board of Health (which had record of his diabetes) asked Jonathan to give some presentations about his diabetes to Community Health Representatives and nurses. He agreed, but only if no one outside the room would find out. In every presentation, to every roomful of healthcare workers, he described his experiences and gave all the insight and information that he could—but asked that each person in the room keep his condition confidential. Secrecy was so much work.

After the fourth presentation, he went to hockey practice. A few hours later, on the way home, he dropped his heavy equipment bag on the sidewalk, pulled out his cellphone, and posted on Facebook that he, Jonathan Linton, had diabetes.

There was no going back. Now, everyone knew.

His hockey team, it turned out, didn't actually care. If he was still the best enforcer around, if he still struck fear into the opposing team, it didn't matter. His girlfriend, who had known for a while but kept the secret, also didn't care. If he treated her well, what did it matter?

What was more surprising was the response of a high school teacher who himself had diabetes: "You know," the teacher said one day, "We diabetics shouldn't play hockey. It's too rough."

It was all Jonathan could do not to laugh. He didn't mean to be rude but he had gone for two years without medication or insulin because of his exercise regime. The exercise had brought his blood sugar levels down. At first, Jonathan thought, *Well, I can't really bother with this guy too much anymore.* The *Aha!* moment came a little later. If a high school teacher, an educated educator with plenty of experience in diabetes, believed something so completely false about the disease, it was time to start talking about diabetes.

Nowadays, Jonathan works as a CHR for the Cree Board of Health. He loves the work. It reminds him to take care of his own health, and he's able to meet people and help them out. He talks about diabetes easily now, and to anyone who wants to hear about it. Just last week, he gave an interview in Cree on CBC radio. He's finishing up high school on the side through homeschooling. His girlfriend, Heather Hughboy, is pregnant; he's getting ready to be a dad and to play more hockey. And to hunt. He's killed porcupine, bear, beaver, caribou, and more—but still no moose.

22

The Story of Anja Diamond* of Nemaska

THE LIFE of Anja (pronounced An-ya) Diamond had not been an easy one, but she had always been able to get rid of stress. Even when she was a young kid, she was an athlete. She played basketball, volleyball, badminton, hockey, soccer, Frisbee, track-and-field, and did pretty much any dry-land sport that came her way. She kept it up after she moved out of her mom's house to be on her own, and she kept it up after she got married. So, whenever bad things happened (and they happened a lot), or when relationships in her life weren't exactly positive (and they often weren't), or even when she just had too much to do and not enough time to do it, she went to the gym and played whatever sport was going on there as hard as she could. The stress and anxiety ran off her body along with the sweat, and she went home and had a good sleep.

One day, in 1996, Anja was playing basketball—she was point guard—and lunged forward to get the ball away from the other team when she felt her knee give out. She collapsed, then picked herself up, signalled for a substitute player to finish the game, and limped off the court. The next day, she went to the clinic and learned

Names and details in this story have been changed to protect identities.

ANJA DIAMOND

her knee was damaged. With time, it healed and she went back to her active life and forgot about the injury.

A few years later, in 2002, Anja was diagnosed with pre-diabetes in a routine blood test, but even that was no big deal: she was so active that her blood sugar levels remained steady and she did not develop diabetes.

The next year, the old knee injury started bothering her. One thing led to another, and soon she was in the operating theatre having surgery. With a few weeks of post-surgery rehab exercises, the knee healed again and Anja went back to the gym, back to her sports—but this time running wasn't the same as it had been before. She could run, sure, but now it was work instead of pleasure. Now it sometimes hurt. Now she was always conscious of how she placed her foot so as not to twist the knee again. Without even realizing, she began exercising less. And with less activity, her pre-diabetes quickly developed into type 2 diabetes. The doctor said she had to start taking pills.

That's when stresses really began to pile up. Anja's sister died suddenly in her early 30s. She had lived with their mom and had taken care of their handicapped brother while their mom was at work, and now Anja's mom was going to have to look after him alone, while also holding down her job. Then Anja's husband started having some unexpected troubles that heaped extra pressure on both of them. There were other things too, like bad memories from her youth that she couldn't stop thinking about. And making it all worse was the fact that she couldn't really talk to anyone about any of it: if she did, then whatever she had said would be used against her in some way. It seemed that every waking minute of every day, Anja was anxious, obsessing about the unfairness of things that had happened to her, and stressed about making sure they wouldn't happen again. She began to experience panic attacks and eventually developed depression.

At least some of the troubles could be managed. Anja, along with her husband, moved back into her mom's house. That way, she wouldn't have to worry about her mom taking care of her brother alone—all three of them could do it—and together, they could grieve the loss of Anja's sister. It worked out just fine. They stayed with her mom, and, every couple of years Anja went to Ottawa to study.

As for the diabetes pills, well. Anja hated taking pills. If she did something that she hated that much, she'd get stressed out even more, so, most of the time, she didn't bother.

At college, Anja studied Aboriginal Studies, Business Accounting, and Community Studies. A classmate asked her once if the James Bay Cree still lived in teepees and cooked outside over open fires. Anja tried not to show her surprise at the question. She kept a straight face and said, politely, "No. We live in houses and cook on stoves that are powered with electricity. Our refrigerators and televisions and computers are also powered with electricity. Sometimes we go into the bush for a few weeks and then we go back home. Our community isn't very different from a small town here, except that it's a lot prettier outside."

Later that term, in a survival skills course out in the bush, Anja realized that she already knew the course material. She had known for years how to live in teepees and cook outside and how to live well in the bush. She could have taught the course. To her classmates from the South it was all new. They couldn't get their teepees to stand upright (it was kind of funny to watch them try), they had no idea where to look for wood or how to make kindling, and they could hardly even start fires properly. Then the food they cooked over the open flame was so awful the dogs wouldn't have eaten it, and they would have poisoned themselves with the wrong berries and leaves if the teacher hadn't been there to correct them. Anja realized then that her classmates didn't understand what her life had been like, and she didn't really understand theirs either.

But many people did understand some of the other difficult things she had gone through. In her Community Studies courses there were people, both professors and students, from both the South and the North, who understood exactly what those parts of her life had been like. They had struggled through some of the same unfair situations, and they had ideas for how she could cope. Also, her courses required her to go through intensive therapy sessions that were often difficult, but in them Anja started to address her feelings and to really know herself, know who she was—and to realize she wasn't trapped by the unfairness of life at all. She couldn't change the past, nobody could, but she could do things to make her life better now and in the future. She came away from her studies still having anxiety, but also having some tools for managing it.

As for those diabetes pills. Every now and then she took one. She was still exercising, though not as much as she once had, and it was keeping her blood sugar levels in check. But she could feel that something was wrong with her body. She was so shaky and weak sometimes, and anxiety could cripple her; did healthy people feel like this? And that blindingly sharp pain in her gut— what was that?

That blinding pain in her gut, she found out after a CT scan, was a hernia. At some point, she didn't know when, she had strained and twisted so severely that some of her intestine had slipped through her abdominal muscle wall and was being pinched. Aside from the pain, the hernia threatened to infect. Anja needed surgery.

She thought back to her knee operation. Her blood sugar levels had been uneven after the surgery and she didn't want that to happen again. So, in the weeks before the hernia operation, Anja went back to the gym and tried to get as fit as she had once been. She was still an athlete; she just needed to be in better shape. But the hernia pain stunned her. She couldn't exercise at all. It hurt so much that she sometimes vomited, and, when that happened, her blood pressure jumped so high that she ended up in the local emergency room. The people there would med-evac her south to bring the blood pressure down. After three or four of these vomiting-high blood pressure episodes, the nurse told her not go to the gym anymore. When the surgery finally happened, it was a relief.

After her hernia surgery, Anja was supposed to rest without exercising for a few weeks while the incision healed and then start once more to exercise gently and strengthen her abdominal muscles. She could hardly wait to be active again. She had felt so good when she could just exercise her worries away, so capable when she could move and run easily. But when the few weeks of recovery were up and she returned to the gym, the blinding pain in her gut came back right away, almost as bad as it had ever been. Even a walk hurt and she would have to stop and rest every few minutes.

This time, it turned out that the pain came from ovarian cysts. The doctor said then that she ought not to exercise as she once had. No team sports, no weights, no running nor even walking long distances, nothing whatsoever that would cause strain. She could swim, he said—but she was afraid of water. As for her diabetes, she was supposed to control it with pills and diet alone.

Now, Anja spent her days sitting. At work she sat. At home she sat. When she was out with her friends, she sat. And with all the sitting, she became less and less fit. The old hernia pain began to flare again, her blood sugar began to climb, and her diabetes began to get worse. More than ever, she was shaky and weak and felt as if something inside of her was very wrong.

She found ways to make her day-to-day life better. For instance, clothing with wide elastic that pressed into her waist reduced the pain in her abdomen. But sometimes it was difficult to help herself. She had always thought of herself as an athlete, as a person who could and would control diabetes without pills or insulin, with exercise alone. How could she do that if she wasn't allowed to exercise, nor even to walk? And if she felt so tired and weak as she always did these days.

And then came another major surgery to remove the ovary that was covered in cysts, followed by a minor skin surgery. With each successive surgery, her blood sugar became more difficult to manage. In the weeks before the last surgery, it climbed so high that the doctors almost didn't go through with the operation. In the end, they decided to do it anyways, and, afterwards her blood sugar level was higher still—almost double what it had been before. The doctors had little choice but to inject insulin into her body to bring the blood sugar down, one kind of insulin into her arm and another kind into her stomach. For three days in a row, they repeated the treatment, and, finally, her blood sugar calmed down.

The doctors put her on an insulin trial then. For a week, while they watched and coached her technique, Anja filled the needle and injected herself with insulin, morning and evening.

To Anja's great surprise, after the one-week insulin trial she felt much better. The difference was like night and day, like summer and winter. She had more energy, she felt happier and had much less anxiety, and she was even able to move more easily. She had never had a medication that had really helped before. Well, she hadn't taken her diabetes pills regularly, that was true, but one reason she hadn't taken them was that any medication she had taken in the years before hadn't really helped.

Anja recovered from the surgery. The insulin had made a genuine difference, so she kept injecting it, morning and evening. Every time she had to pierce her skin, either to test her blood sugar or to inject insulin, a small part of her felt like she was making a huge personal sacrifice and another small part felt that needing insulin at all was a personal failure. But the relief at feeling so much better soon outweighed the negativity.

She began studying diabetes like she had studied Business Accounting, to get a grasp on how it worked. In her eating, she had always tried to eat foods the Canada Food Guide recommended—that had been fine before—but it wasn't diabetes-specific. She worked with a diabetes specialist nurse to understand how a body with diabetes reacted to different kinds of food, and the precise insulin calculations that specific foods required. It was news to her that certain foods affected blood sugar more than others, she had never known that eating too much was unhealthy, and she had never heard that some foods (like sugars) were actually toxic if you ate too much of them. Her anxieties, she had always thought, were because of her fixation on unfair things that had happened to her. She was completely surprised to find out that anxiety was also a symptom of hypoglycemia (low blood sugar). She had never realized that eating breakfast was actually important to maintaining healthy blood sugar levels. Anja was like a kid in elementary school, learning about food for the very first time. She didn't much crave sugar or junk food, so changing her diet wasn't difficult—but there were so many changes she had to make.

Anja eats mostly traditional food now. She has an arrangement with the hunters in her family: they keep her freezer full, and she does the cleaning and butchering. They all help each other out. She has also begun to talk with family members about diabetes. It runs in her family, but it was never something that people talked about at home. Anja is changing that.

Now that Anja understands more about diabetes, she has moved on to research something else: gastric bypass surgery. Gastric bypass is an extreme operation in which surgeons create a small thumb-sized pouch in the stomach to receive food, closing off the rest of the stomach, and then they attach the small intestine to the pouch. After getting this surgery, people can eat only tiny amounts of food—as much as the thumb-sized pouch can hold—for the rest of their lives. Never again, not even once, can they eat a big meal. It's a drastic and permanent way-of-life shift. Anja is considering gastric bypass because other people who have had it have seen dramatic improvements in their diabetes. She would much rather exercise her way to diabetes control, but her doctor still warns her not to exercise, and she doesn't have many other options for helping herself. Secretly, she thinks gastric bypass might reduce the pain in her abdomen and allow her to be active again; she misses exercise much more than she would ever miss food.

More and more, Anja thinks of diabetes and Cree health in terms of responsibility. Colonization changed so many aspects of Cree life and health. It forced people into settlements and residential schools and it introduced diets rife with packaged foods. But some changes came about because Cree folks switched to driving cars and SUVs and ATVs instead of walking everywhere like they used to do, to buying packaged foods instead of filling the freezer with hunted game and fish, to sitting in front of televisions and computers too long every day. Even the James Bay Hydroelectric Project—it was another brutal upheaval forced upon the Cree, but along the way they made some choices and had some influence on how the Project turned out in the end. Anja wonders if some of the increase in diabetes and other illnesses has come about because of choices people make that are not always healthy choices, even if those choices are only the very smallest part of the big picture.

Taking responsibility for these choices, however small, is important to Anja for a simple reason: when she focussed on injustices in her past, she felt powerless, and that made the injustices feel worse. But when she took responsibility for her own choices and for her own health, she was able to focus on the future and all its possibilities, and she was able to do things that made her healthier. Anja wonders if better living for the James Bay Cree costs something—and if that cost might be taking responsibility for it and making the choices to build a healthier life.

Stories We Heard Along the Way: Tidbits

In years past, the artists and craftspeople who did traditional beadwork always made an intentional error in their creations (usually one wrong bead) to show humility to the Great Spirit and to recognize that her creations were always perfect.

•

Even the social workers say that the Meechum store in Mistissini is one of the most important social welfare organizations in Eeyou Istchee. The store extends lines of credit to people in great need, it matches monetary donations made to the food bank, it sells groceries to the food bank at wholesale prices, and, in countless other ways, it contributes to the health of the Cree Nation of Mistissini. Over the years, the Meechum store has built such loyalty that the Northern Store couldn't make it in Mistissini, even though it had lower prices on some products.

•

Climate change is afoot. In recent years, polar bears have been seen as far south as Waskaganish.

•

When Nemaska was relocated to its current sandy location, the Province of Québec sent up soil scientists to confirm that the soil was stable enough for houses. Teepees, lighter and portable to begin with, had never caused problems. Unfortunately, the soil scientists didn't get it quite right and some of the houses began to sink into the soil. A different design had to be used for the newer houses.

•

A representative of the Cree Board of Health travelled to Montréal to present information showing that diabetes was more prevalent in the communities most affected by the James Bay Hydroelectric Project. Sûreté du Québec informed him then that threats had been made against him—and the threats were so severe that he would need bodyguards at the meeting.

•

A number of storytellers in this book spoke of never seeing a fence before they went to residential school. At residential school, in the middle of a perfectly good open space, someone had erected posts and/or wire. The storytellers talked about staring at it, trying to figure out why someone would want to build anything that made crossing an open space so difficult. Then they learned that the fence was there to contain them, and if they climbed over it or crossed it in any way they would be punished.

23

The Story of Angela Etapp of Waskaganish

IN FEBRUARY 1998, Angela Etapp was in Ottawa, on her way to catch a bus and go to class at Algonquin College where she was studying Aboriginal Studies. The weather was terrible. Freezing rain, wet enough to penetrate her coat and cold enough to slick up everything. Not just a few millimetres of ice like Ottawa so often got, but four or five inches of it. She'd never seen anything like it.

She stepped as gingerly as she could—and didn't get very far before she wiped out on the ice. Nine months pregnant, she didn't want to take too many risks, so she carefully got to her feet, turned around, and went back home.

On the radio in her kitchen, they were calling it The Great Ice Storm of 1998. Angela took off her coat and was hanging it up when she felt something else altogether: a long deep cramp from the top of her abdomen to the bottom of her thighs, and a plug of mucus came out of her. It was strange, unlike anything she had felt before. She probably needed to lie down. And then the cramp passed and everything went back to normal. They were beginning to talk on the radio about the damage and blackouts the ice storm was causing.

A while later, she had another long cramp from the top of her abdomen to the bottom of her thighs. She picked up the phone and called her clinic in Waskaganish and told them what was happening.

"Well, I can't be sure without seeing you," the lady on the phone said, "but it sounds like you might be going into labour. Can you get to a hospital?"

Angela looked around her apartment—she had meant to tidy up today. Oh well. Another cramp came just then. She waited for it to pass, and walked into the other room and told her boyfriend what was happening.

He looked at her strangely. "Labour? Are you sure?"

"That's what the lady on the phone said. I kinda believe her."

Angela called the Ottawa hospital for an ambulance and told them where she was.

"Uh, ma'am, I'm sorry but we can't treat you in Ontario. You have a Québec health card. You have to go to a Québec hospital."

"But this really hurts!" Angela said. "You're a few kilometres away and there's an ice storm outside."

"Can you take a cab to a Québec hospital?" they asked.

Angela waited for another long cramp to pass. A cab cost too much. She had only thirty dollars. Maybe she could take the bus.

She talked it over with her boyfriend and they realized that the bus would take 45 minutes at least. And, in the storm, probably more. They had no choice. Another long cramp came just then, and her boyfriend called a cab. They would have to give the driver all of their money and hope it was enough. And also hope no other expenses came up.

Angela's boyfriend told the driver to take them to the nearest hospital in Hull. The driver went as quickly as he could on the iced streets. All through the everlasting ride, he kept looking back at her anxiously and talking to her boyfriend.

"Is she okay?" he asked, as the car skidded sideways a bit.

"We think she's going into labour."

"Look at her!" the driver said. "She's not *going into* anything. She's been at it for a while! She gonna be able to hold the kid in?"

Angela was in so much pain that she hardly noticed them.

The receptionist at the hospital yawned, barely glanced at Angela, and wheeled her into the waiting room to wait with everyone else who wanted to see a doctor. The cramps were coming faster and faster and each was more intense than the one before.

Finally, another woman in the waiting room walked up to the reception desk and pointed at Angela.

"Excuse me," she said. "I think that lady is in labour. I've had babies. It's very messy. If you make her have a baby in the waiting room, you'll have a lot of cleaning up to do."

The receptionist looked up, reluctantly, expelled a huge sigh, and signalled an orderly to wheel Angela into an exam room. Angela changed into the paper gown and the cramps just kept right on coming. Twenty minutes later, a young doctor strolled in.

"What seems to be the problem?" he asked.

And Angela bore down into the longest, deepest cramp yet and kicked out her legs until it finally stopped.

"Shit!!" he shouted out into the hallway. "That's a contraction! This woman is in labour!" He checked her quickly and shouted again. "Shit! She's fully dilated!"

An older doctor came running then. He lifted Angela's gown and took a look. And then he looked at her sweaty, exhausted face.

"First baby?" he asked.

"Yes."

"Well, you're not just in labour, honey. The baby's crowning. You're about to deliver. But we don't deliver babies in this hospital, you see. Your baby's not allowed to be born here and you're not allowed to give birth here. You have to go either to an Ottawa hospital if you're from Ontario, or to the Gatineau hospital if you're from Québec."

Surely, it was the stupidest thing that Angela had ever heard. In the history of babies, had there ever been a baby who researched hospital policy before it was born? But her body was splitting and she was in no position to argue. The doctor called the ambulance to rush Angela to the Gatineau hospital.

Everything inside of her said it was the baby's time to be born. All the way to Gatineau, Angela tried not to push it out until they got to the right hospital, but not pushing was the hardest thing she had ever done. The paramedic in the ambulance had her hand between Angela's legs, on the baby's head, trying to help Angela keep the baby inside. Neither of them noticed the storm outside.

"Mon Dieu, mon Dieu," the paramedic said. "J'espère que vous n'allez pas l'avoir ici. Pas ici!" *My god, please don't have the baby here. Not here!*

As soon as they pulled up to the door of the hospital, the paramedic pulled away her hand.

"Okay," she said—and there, on the gurney, just inside the hospital door, baby Aaron slid out in a mess of amniotic fluid and began to holler his arrival to the world.

Angela and her boyfriend couldn't stop laughing.

The next six months were exhausting and wonderful. Aaron was a healthy, giggly baby with a good appetite and very strong lungs. Angela wasn't feeling quite herself just yet, and her house wasn't as tidy as she liked it to be, but that, she thought, was to be expected with a new baby.

And then, one night, Aaron went to sleep in his crib and never woke up. He died of Sudden Infant Death Syndrome (SIDS) just before his six-month birthday.

Angela's time with her beautiful son was up.

Her world fell apart. Nothing was worse than the death of a child, the psychologists said so. During her pregnancy, she had had gestational diabetes, the diabetes that pregnant women get and that usually goes away once the baby is born. Now, she was tired and thirsty all the time, but her body, still adjusting to childbirth, had to adjust to the death of an infant. For sure, that's all it was.

Two months after Aaron was buried, she went to the clinic for a check-up. The doctor said that her gestational diabetes had not gone away after childbirth. It had become type 2 diabetes and it would never go away.

Angela nodded at the news but it didn't really sink in. Her baby had died. Why would she bother to think about diabetes? Why would diabetes matter at all?

The doctor kept talking. She might feel okay now, he said, but she would see the effects of diabetes on her body in ten or fifteen years, when her organs would start to fail. Certainly, he said, she would die young.

Angela went home to Waskaganish.

How could she have type 2 diabetes? It was an old person's disease and she was only 22. Her grandparents had had diabetes but they had never really talked to her about it. They had lived far away in Senneterre, and, any time she had seen them, she hadn't thought to ask. She knew that her grandfather had lost both feet to diabetes, and her grandmother had had a heart attack because of it, but neither of them were just 22 years old.

Whatever. She was tired, needed a nap. Grieving moms needed sleep. Some days she needed so much sleep she wouldn't see the light of day. She'd go to bed at night and sleep all the way through until the next evening. When she was awake, she had a wedding to plan. Her boyfriend's parents had suggested they get married so that they could heal from the death of their son together. And she was pregnant again. She didn't really have time to think about diabetes.

In August of 2000, with another month to go before her second baby was due, Angela went to visit friends in Val-d'Or. While she was there, she got a phone call from a friend in Waskaganish who told her that her husband was at home in their brand new house in Waskaganish—with another woman.

Angela tried to stay calm, but her body knew she was upset. Her blood pressure jumped way up, and right away she had one of those long, deep cramps from the top of her abdomen to the bottom of her thighs. This time, she knew she was in labour.

The friends she was staying with rushed her to the hospital. Immediately the doctor saw that something was wrong because her blood pressure was so high.

"I just found out my husband is sleeping with another woman in my house, my *brand new* house," she said. "I'm trying to stay calm, but it's not working!"

"Well, ma'am, you're going to have your baby tonight. It's early, but you're far enough along that the baby should be okay. As long as we can bring your blood pressure down."

They gave her an epidural analgesia, a type of pain medication that's put directly into the spinal cord region so that women in labour can't feel the contractions, and her second son, as beautiful as the first, was born in the morning, a year and five days after the death of baby Aaron.

Angela cried for an hour, she was so happy for him. And so upset at her husband. With a new baby in her arms and no one to share the experience with, she felt euphoric—and utterly alone. From that night on, Angela always had to watch her blood pressure carefully because it would jump right away at the first sign of stress.

And from that night on, she hovered over the crib, watching the baby sleep, and thinking of her first baby, Aaron. Until her son was a year old, she stayed up late and woke early to watch him sleep. As long as she was watching, he would not die of SIDS, and so she watched him every minute that she could. And when the next baby came along, she did the same.

In November of 2002, Angela's marriage came to an end. Eventually, she moved on with another man who loved her and her boys, and altogether they built a noisy, happy home. In spring and summer every year, they headed out onto the land where they hunted and fished and filled the freezer. They spent as much time out there as they could. When they were in town, she worked for the Cree Board of Health as an administrator.

In August 2003, Angela's boyfriend was leaving for work at a camp just outside of Waskaganish. Angela gave him a big goodbye hug—he would be gone for just a few days—and he climbed into the truck and looked back at her as she waved. She was supposed to drive to work then, but as soon as she slid behind the wheel she decided to bend the rules a bit and follow the truck. She would say goodbye to him one more time.

She buckled her seat belt around her big belly—she was pregnant with her fourth child—and set off after the truck. She rounded a big bend in the road and saw his truck up ahead. And also saw a big ten-wheeler truck turning right in front of her. There was no way she could stop in time.

Instinctively, she put back her head and closed her eyes. "Oh Jesus," she whispered.

Her car skidded under the ten-wheeler and jammed there, everything above the engine hood sheared right off.

But Angela was somewhere else, somewhere she had never been. There were quite a few people. The whole place was full of light, a white light brighter than the sun. She was walking towards the people, and at her side was someone about nine feet tall, wearing white robes and going in the same direction. Two people were walking towards her. A guy in a white gown with a purple sash across the chest and a little boy beside him. She recognized the boy right away: it was her late son Aaron. He was happy and full of life. Then someone was calling out her name behind her—she turned around to see who it was, then turned back to her son once more, but Aaron and the man beside him were gone.

Angela woke then. Her car seat had done something very unusual. The mechanism that keeps the seat upright had suddenly unlatched and her seat had dropped instantly all the way back. If it hadn't, if it had stayed upright like the seat beside her, her head would have been cut off. She had a broken collarbone and a scratch or two. Otherwise, she was fine and the baby inside of her was fine.

But she had had a glimpse of her firstborn who had died. A gift. And he was okay.

The worst stresses of childbirth and infancy and a struggling marriage were behind her. She still thought about baby Aaron and what she had seen the day of the car accident, and she took care of her kids and new husband, but now she also had a bit of time to think about her own health. She loved food—poutine, salad, cheeseburgers, bannock, cereal, vegetables, you name it. She loved even thinking about food. She had always been an organized sort of person—she had to be in her job—so it seemed natural to her to begin keeping track of what she ate and how much on a spreadsheet. She also kept track of how much diabetes medication she took, of how many minutes she had spent exercising, and what kind of exercise she had done. And then, since she was recording all this stuff anyways, she began recording her blood sugar levels on the same spreadsheet. Sometimes, she even drew her data on a bar or line graph.

There, with all the information laid out on a tidy graph in front of her, it didn't take long at all to see that her blood sugar jumped suddenly every time she ate certain foods (pasta, bannock, cereal), and then she would have to inject a whole lot of insulin. Other foods (game, vegetables) kept her blood sugar levels even and healthy or even brought them down. And other foods were somewhere in between; brown bread pushed up her sugar levels but not nearly as much as white bread did. Sometimes, with traditional foods and after a day of walking or cross-country skiing, she didn't have to take any insulin at all. She began to modify her eating a little, and she began to exercise even more, partly to feel better—and partly to make for nice even bars on her graph and spreadsheet.

Every so often, one of her sons would speak longingly of something he had eaten at someone else's house. Did she know about white bread? And that you could buy it at the Northern? Shouldn't they try a little more of that at home on their table? And did she know that some chocolate bars had peanuts in them, and that peanuts were healthy? She would smile, feed him brown bread or vegetables, and start talking about health until her son rolled his eyes and left the room, convinced his mother was hopeless.

Seventeen years after her diagnosis and seven years after she began taking diabetes seriously, Angela had many years of data saved in spreadsheets on her computer. A nice even chart without any blood sugar jumps and dives was still what motivated her to eat carefully and to exercise regularly. She had signed up for the 100-kilometre walk. The doctor who had said that her organs would begin shutting down years ago couldn't have been more wrong.

Last year, for the first time, Angela attended the Waskaganish community memorial service for everyone who has passed away. It's an annual event in which the whole community comes together, and everyone grieves and remembers their loved ones and celebrates the lives they lived. Angela celebrated and grieved her eldest, baby Aaron. She stood there, in the midst of all the mourners, remembering all the good times she had had in her six months with him and how happy and loved he had looked in that other place in the light.

She felt closure and peace.

She left the ceremony and went home to her other kids. Two of them had a hockey game that night and she wanted to watch them play. And after that, they were all barbecuing moose for dinner.

24

The Story of Joey Blacksmith of Waswanipi

ON A FRIDAY evening in May of 2014, after a long day of fishing on Lake Waswanipi, Joey Blacksmith drove his boat back to shore. When the boat hit gravel, he hopped onto the beach, grabbed the bow to pull it in, and felt something shoot into his left foot. He had probably stepped on a piece of garbage, no big deal. He secured the boat, picked up the string of fish, and headed for the campsite. He and his family ate flame-roasted fish for dinner and lingered around the fire for a while, then he crawled into his bed, and he fell into the deep sleep that comes when you're out on the land.

Saturday was another beautiful day of fishing with the family, followed by dinner, an evening around a snapping fire, and sleep.

On Sunday morning, Joey woke before his family. It was the day to leave his wife and kids at the camp and drive down to Montréal. He was taking Master of Business Administration courses at McGill, and classes started on Monday. His foot felt a little hot, though. He crawled out of the tent, careful not to wake his wife, and hobbled over to a big log. He took a look at his foot. It was swollen. The slightest pressure from his fingers burned and the pain was most intense right where he had stepped on something the other night. But, even in the bright sunlight, he couldn't see if a sliver or anything else had slipped under the skin.

Soon everyone woke, they had breakfast, and he headed out.

As he drove, the pain in his foot got worse, so Joey stopped in at the clinic in Waswanipi and the doctor applied a cream. "When you get to Montréal," he said to Joey, "get it checked again. And drive safely."

Joey settled in behind the wheel and began to think about what he usually thought about on his the long drive to Montréal: the business he was building. He had bought an outfitter's camp half an hour outside of Waswanipi on his family's traditional trap-line land. He was turning it into a cultural site. He would market all over the world and bring international tourists to Eeyou Istchee. He would erect teepees and cabins, hire local Cree people to be cooks and fishing guides and hunting guides and maintenance personnel and trail tenders, and he would offer tours and excursion packages, even in winter. They would have to buy a fleet of snowmobiles. Maybe a snowmobile company would give them a discount if he bought twenty. The thing was, the more Joey thought about his outfitter's camp, the more his foot hurt.

He concentrated. They'd need snowshoes too. The light-weight metal ones? Or traditional wood-and-sinew ones? Metal ones needed less maintenance, but people might pay for the opportunity to use traditional snowshoes and having them made could employ more Cree people. Eventually, if business exploded, he could add a casino or golf resort, but if business was slow, he'd keep it small and intimate. That'd be nice too. His business profs said to plan for both and consid–

CRAP!! That foot really hurt!

He concentrated. The outfitter's camp would provide jobs for local people who hated being on social assistance. Joey was already sending future employees to take courses they would need at the Waswanipi Vocational *his foot!* College. Most of them loved it. They loved studying *his foot!* material that would be useful and that used the traditional knowledge *his foot!* they already had—

Joey pulled over. He couldn't think about his outfitter's camp. He could hardly think about the road. The only thing that mattered was relieving the pain in his foot.

He was 60 kilometres from home. There was no way he would get all the way to Montréal with this pain. He would have to miss the first day of class, but he really couldn't do this.

Joey wheeled the truck around and drove back to Waswanipi. His own house was empty—his family was still in the bush—so he pulled into his mom's driveway and hobbled to the door. He let himself in and walked straight to the couch, where he collapsed on his mom's sofa and put his foot up.

The next morning, Joey's foot was at least three times the size it should have been. No sock would fit around it. It didn't even look like a foot and the pain was unbelievable. Any time he put it down, he could feel infection sloshing about inside.

Something was seriously wrong. Pain or no pain, he had to get to Montréal.

He hopped out to his truck and tried again to drive to Montréal. He made no attempt to think about his outfitter's camp. He put all of his mental effort into driving fifty kilometres. Then he pulled over, lay down on the seat of his truck and raised his foot to relieve the pressure. After fifteen minutes of rest, he drove another fifty kilometres. At one point he got so used to the pain that he drove almost a hundred kilometres without stopping but, still, a drive that usually took him no more than seven hours took over eleven. By the time he got to the city, it was too late for the hospital. He went to his place in Montréal and crashed—but the pain was so intense he didn't sleep all night.

The next morning, hardly able to talk from pain, he drove straight to the hospital.

The doctors and nurses were even more alarmed than he was. Right away they gave him a shot for the pain. Then they hooked him up to an IV to shrink the swelling and X-rayed the foot. Sure enough, a tiny metal shard had slipped inside and was causing infection. They brought over a tray of instruments, cut the foot open and extracted the shard, doused everything with antibiotics, and said a bunch of stuff, Joey hardly noticed. That first day in the hospital, the only thing that really mattered was that the pain had finally stopped.

The next six days were a nightmare of their own. Joey was in much less pain, and he had given up on the first week of classes, but his toes were turning black. The doctors thought gangrene was setting in and they would have to amputate two toes at least. If they didn't, the gangrene would spread and Joey would lose his whole foot. Maybe even his leg.

How was this possible?

Joey had always been an athlete—hockey, track and field, basketball, all that stuff. And he had been the Youth Grand Chief of Eeyou Istchee for five years. He had envisioned all sorts of things for his own future and for the future of the Cree Nation of Waswanipi, but he had never, in his entire life, thought of himself as a guy who might lose his toes or his foot or his leg!

The doctor mentioned that Joey's blood sugar level was 13— he had diabetes. That was news, but not terribly surprising. He'd been tested for it a few times because diabetes ran in his family, but none of the doctors or nurses had noted anything unusual in his blood sugar levels. Or if they had, they hadn't told him. But amputation was something that happened to people way down the road, after they'd had diabetes for years and years and their blood sugar levels climbed above 25. Amputation wasn't something that happened because of a single misstep on a springtime fishing trip. It wasn't something that happened to a young guy with a blood sugar of 13.

Was it?

As soon as he was able, Joey posted everything on Facebook: his misshapen foot, his crazy drive to Montréal, his toes turning black, his diabetes diagnosis, his possible amputation. All of Eeyou Istchee knew who he was from his days as Youth Grand Chief, and support flooded in. People thinking of him, praying for him, texting him, and posting on Facebook so that he wouldn't feel alone.

A doctor bustled into his room. "We're gonna try one last thing, Joey. We want to inject your foot with iodine that's been mixed with dye. Then we're gonna X-ray it again. If even a tiny amount of dye travels to the tips of your two black toes, then we'll know there's a wee bit of circulation there and we can throw everything at it to help it along. But if there's no circulation, then the toes are already dead and they'll have to come off immediately."

Joey posted that bit of information on Facebook too, and then he signalled the doctor to inject him.

On the X-ray, they saw, in each black toe, a skinny tributary of iodine snake its way to the tips. His toes could be saved.

The thing about sitting in a hospital—it gives you time to think. The more Joey thought about it, the more this situation sucked. People in his family had died of diabetes. Would he be next? What of his Joey-the-athlete and Joey-the-leader and Joey-the-hunter-trapper identities? His kids thought of their dad as a healthy guy. Now he'd be Joey-the-diabetic, Joey-the-sick-guy-who-has-to-take-pills-with-dinner, let's all feel sorry for Poor Joey. Poor Joey is not who he was. It made him grumpy.

He and his family had just moved back to Eeyou Istchee. They had lived in Montréal for three years so his wife could finish her Bachelor's degree at university. They had adjusted to city life. With restaurants and bakeries everywhere you looked, with watermelon (Joey's favourite fruit) all year-round, with all kinds of wonderful new foods to try, their diet had changed. And Joey and his wife had abandoned the sports and activities that had been part of life in Waswanipi. In the city, where everything was spread out, Joey's free time went to driving his kids to dance lessons and after-school activities and helping them adjust to city life and to French-language schooling. There was no time for hockey and no need for the rigor of chopping wood. By the end of three years, when Joey poked his gut, it was kind of soft. He had less energy than he had had before moving to Montréal. Just three years of city life, and here he was, in his hometown again—but with diabetes.

Joey had probably been predisposed to diabetes because it ran in his family. But three years of inactivity and hello diabetes? That was something to think about. During his time in Cree youth leadership, he'd noticed that the healthiest families were those living on the land. He had heard of quite a few elders whose health problems—from cancer to diabetes to mental illness—had improved dramatically when they returned to the land and to traditional foods and activities. That was kind of cool, but what did it mean? So much of Cree identity came from life on the land. His cultural site business was about that.

But in truth, even on the land they were not always doing things in traditional ways. In truth, they were doing a whole lot of sitting. Even hunting these days often happened on the cushioned seats of snowmobiles and four-wheelers. It was too easy.

On his seventh morning in the hospital, the doctors finally had Joey's foot situation under control and they sent him home. For a long time yet, he would be on antibiotics to bring down the swelling. And he'd be managing diabetes for the rest of his life.

That made him grumpy too.

Joey had a friend, about the same age, and who had lost a leg to diabetes and had had other diabetes-related surgeries. Even with all his surgeries, no one thought of him as sick and no one felt sorry for him. He did it all: public speaking, moose hunting, working full-time, parenting, volunteering all over the place, you name it.

He was one inspiring guy. About ten days after Joey's diagnosis, when he was still feeling grumpy, his friend texted him.

"Heard about your diagnosis. Bummer. But you can't mope, your body can't take it. Get moving. Help yourself. With diabetes, the doctors can do only so much. Bummer, but get off your butt."

Joey put down his phone and looked at his still-attached toes and otherwise healthy body. Really, what did he have to complain about?

In the next three weeks, Joey spoke to crowds three times about diabetes. He learned quickly that diabetes was a serious Cree problem—by now probably every Eeyou Istchee family was affected—and it needed Cree solutions. Joey was new at this and didn't yet know what Cree solutions would look like, but he could begin by going public. Many Cree people with diabetes didn't admit they had it. Some couldn't even bring themselves to take their pills. Shame just made everything worse. The way to take down shame was to talk about diabetes publicly.

And there was the problem of day-to-day changes at home now that diabetes was in the house. One of Joey's friends had taken a diabetic cooking course. Joey called him for food advice and went online for exercise ideas. New food habits, new routines, new things to research, new exercise schedules. New problems to solve.

Joey's kids were not thrilled. They especially protested their dad's new enthusiasm for exercise. What was the point of exercise, they said, when *they* didn't have diabetes? What was the point of it when sitting in front of a gaming console was so much more interesting? Still, Joey forced them to do it. Diabetes management and prevention would be a lifelong uphill battle, but families everywhere across Eeyou Istchee were in the same position.

It wouldn't be easy for any of them.

25

The Story of Coco Simone Chanelle* of Mistissini

SPRING 2009: Coco Simone Chanelle walked into the Sporting Goods store in Mistissini and approached the rack of shotguns along the wall. One by one, she lifted them to her shoulder, sighting along the barrels, feeling for the trigger, making sure the heft and proportions were right for her short arms. A couple of hours later she walked out with a new shotgun—a nice, light .410 gauge—slung across her back. A girl ought to have her own gun.

When Coco was a kid, she wanted to be independent. Her grandmother had grown up in the bush, far from other people. She had lived with her family in a teepee made of skins and wood, her food and medicines had come from the land, and her fuel had come from trees that were chopped down into firewood. She hadn't needed grocery stores nor shopping malls nor the internet nor crowds of friends. She had been self-sufficient.

It must be wonderful, taking care of yourself like that, Coco thought. *To be able to build your own house and chop your own wood and hunt your own food. To not need anyone else. To like who*

*Names and details in this story have been changed to protect identities.

you are enough to enjoy your own company best of all. She wanted to be like that.

She was thinking about her grandmother in high school math class one day. What would her grandmother have done if she had walked through a stand of tamarack and come upon a chalk board of intolerably boring calculus problems? Coco yawned—she had to stay awake another 25 minutes. A boy was watching her yawn and laughing. She smiled back at him. Now there were only 24 minutes left in the class.

Soon Coco's life was full of that boy. She sat beside him in the lunchroom. He cheered her at her broomball games. She spent her free evenings with him and his friends. She graduated from high school, married him, and left her parents' house to move into his family home in another community. She could do her post-secondary schooling by correspondence from there. He was a nice guy and it was a good life. Things would be okay.

As the years passed, her husband's work contracts took him away from home for longer periods of time. He would come home for a few days and then have to leave again.

Coco kept busy. Between pregnancies, she got a Certificate in Office Administration. Between changing diapers, she finished a Diploma in Social Sciences. Between cheering at her kids' broom-ball and hockey tournaments and helping them with homework assignments, she earned a Bachelor of Arts degree in Comparative Literature and History. And when the kids finished high school, she finished her Master of Arts degree in Sociology.

Her husband helped pay the bills. When he saw Coco and the kids, he always treated them well. When he was there, he was a good companion and partner and father. But he was hardly ever there. Coco was raising their daughter and son alone, married only on paper. Years earlier, she had wanted to be independent, but this wasn't quite what she had had in mind.

Winter 2001. Coco ran into the bathroom at work and closed the door behind her. She yanked down her pants. And she scratched and rubbed until the whole area between her legs was raw. Then she looked at her watch: for thirty beautiful seconds, she felt no itch. She was in heaven. And then it came back with a vengeance, hotter and more maddening than before. There could be no doubt. She had *another* vaginal yeast infection.

How could that be? It had been only three weeks since she had finished the prescription for the last infection! She rinsed and dried herself off, put her clothes in order, and went back to her desk. She picked up the phone and dialed the number for the clinic. She wouldn't be able to get any work done until the itch was taken care of.

A few days later, she was back at her desk, staring at the cubicle wall. Again, she was having trouble working. The itching and burning were gone—her clinic visit had taken care of that—but the doctor had blown the bottom out of her world: Coco had had so many yeast infections lately because the balance of bacteria in her body had been upset by uneven blood sugar levels. She had diabetes.

Diabetes! she thought. *What am I going to eat? I'll starve!*

The cubicle wall had no answers for her.

And then she thought, *Oh for heaven's sake. Of all the diabetes symptoms in the world, couldn't I have gotten one less embarrassing than vaginal yeast infections? Like being thirsty or shaky or something?*

The next day, she was calmer. She had had some time to think about the diagnosis and about her relatives with diabetes and to read some of the clinic pamphlets.

People with diabetes still eat. I just have to change the way I eat.

She made lists of foods then—ones she would eat less (starches and sweets) and ones she would eat more (meats and vegetables). She also made lists of exercises she liked to do. For two whole years, she stuck to the lists. She ate carefully and exercised regularly and was one of the lucky ones who could control her diabetes without medication.

And then her personal life interfered.

Summer 2004: The kids were almost grown and Coco began to daydream again about independence out in the bush, about more schooling far away, by herself. The trouble was that a piece of paper said she was married. Attached, not independent. A thought crept into her mind. *What about—divorce?*

From a good guy who treated her well but just wasn't there? People would say that a good mother could never do such a thing. People would say that divorce would damage her kids. Or that their happiness was more important than hers and she should sacrifice more. Or that others had it so much worse and she should just get over herself already. Communities could be so difficult. It wasn't worth it. The best thing to do, Coco decided, was to bear down and try harder to be content in her marriage.

And the kids, her beautiful daughter and handsome son— they were *really* fighting. They used to be such good friends and now they couldn't stand each other. One little thing led to another and then one grudge and then another and the problems accumulated— until finally her son brought charges against her daughter and the police were involved. Coco didn't recognize these angry people. Was this all because of her? If she could force herself to be content in her own marriage, could her kids follow her example and find ways to be content in their relationship with each other?

Coco lay awake at night trying to quell the yearning for independence that gnawed at her ribcage. She jolted awake too early in the morning, her mind grasping for solutions to her kids' warfare. What could she do? Was there something she could say to one of them to make her or him stop hating the other? The anxiety was overwhelming, more than she could cope with, and the more anxious she became, the higher her blood sugar levels climbed. Soon Coco was taking medication for her diabetes. Still she couldn't stop lying awake at night or jolting awake too soon in the morning. Still the family skirmishes continued. And still she wanted out of her marriage.

The diabetes was getting worse—her blood sugar levels were all over the place now, way up at one moment and way down the next. She had become weak and shaky and nervous about holding fragile things for fear she'd break them. Finally, after a day of one shaky spell after another, Coco admitted something she had known inside of herself for a while already: these relationship problems were affecting her health and she could not fix them herself. She didn't have the specialized skills necessary to resolve the conflict between her kids, and she was too exhausted even to think about what to do about the other things bothering her.

She made arrangements to see a psychologist in Montréal. Surely, the psychologist would tell her how to be content in her marriage and how to fix her kids' problems. The psychologist would have the answers. She packed her bags and flew down to Montréal.

The psychologist sessions were not what Coco expected. He didn't coach her in marriage contentment. He didn't give her a single solution to her kids' fighting. But he listened to her and asked hard questions until Coco could see her own answers. That trying harder to be content would never fix her marriage. That she could do nothing about what other people said. They talked because they wanted to, not because of what she did or didn't do, and she could never control their talking so there was no point wasting energy on thinking about it. But facing the problems and taking care of her own happiness—these were things that she could do.

And so she did them. She started with an honest and calm discussion with her husband and admitted that she wanted a divorce. At their own kitchen table, without lawyers or mediators,

Coco and her husband came to a quiet and amicable agreement. They paid off all debts. They treated one another with affection and respect. They filed a joint application for divorce and ended their marriage as friends, without grievances. There were no fights nor custody battles. And Coco's blood sugar levelled out soon after that. It surprised her—this close relationship between her own happiness and her diabetes.

And now for the fighting kids. She hated to admit it, but Coco knew from her work with the psychologist that she was not the problem in her kids' relationship. She was not the one fighting, so she could not fix it. What she could do was make help available to them if they wanted it. If they chose to keep fighting, she would not be able to control it.

She spoke to her son and daughter, one at a time, and both agreed to meet with elders for counselling and with a mediator, a type of therapist who could work with them to untangle the old hard knots of their grudges. Gradually, with time and effort, the kids began to listen to each other and rebuild tolerance and respect for one another. Eventually the charges were dropped.

Fall 2010: Coco and her aunt bought a car and packed some bags and drove across the country all the way to Edmonton, Alberta. They had both enrolled in classes there. Coco's aunt soon got lonely and came back to Québec, but Coco stayed. She had her own apartment, a small one-bedroom place with hardwood floors and an aqua-coloured stove. For the first time in her life, she lived alone. At first, she was apprehensive. What if she wouldn't like her own company? Wouldn't that mean she didn't like herself? Coco had to learn to cook for one person, to do laundry for one person, to schedule a life for one person—it was all new—and she found that she liked her own company best of all.

In the cold winter mornings, when it was forty below, she bundled up and went for long walks. The exercise was good for her diabetes and the prairies had an uncluttered elegance about them that was strangely comforting. She bought books about diabetes and she read them over breakfast and between classes and in the long winter evenings. She learned yoga poses that helped her relax and stay fit. She looked into acupuncture that was supposed to help people manage diabetes. She learned about food labels and how the numbers on the label affected her health. She attended her classes and spoke with her psychologist. She developed a much more positive outlook.

She woke early one day, not from anxiety but because she wanted to go for a walk—and realized that she was healthy. She had diabetes, and she was also healthy. After a year in Alberta, Coco had to return to Québec for work, but her experiment had succeeded. She had moved away from everything she knew and had lived alone, happy, healthy, for an entire year.

She was her grandmother's kin.

Spring 2013: Coco slipped her truck into gear and drove to the grocery store. She bought supplies and loaded them into the truck. She was heading out to her father's trapline, seven hours inland, where she would stay in the bush for a few weeks, hunting small game, learning to live off the land. Then she had would return to town, to her warm house with its electricity and to her work. She would visit her acupuncturist in Montréal, look into setting up her own business, and visit her wonderful kids. She had been doing this—heading out into the bush alone—for a while and had developed many of the skills that her grandmother once had.

She closed the latch on the back of her truck, then swung once more by her house to pick up her clothing and the rest of her gear. And of course her .410 gauge. A girl ought to have her own gun.

26

The Story of Freddie Wapachee of Nemaska

FREDDIE'S dad was a trapper and a hunter who lived in the bush near the shores of Lake Nemaska. Other Nemaska people lived nearby and every few days someone was bound to look in on you, make sure everything was okay. Chop some wood if the woodpile was low. Bring fresh fish on a string or a hunk of moose for the elders who were getting too slow to hunt. Have a cup of tea or talk about the weather. The Cree tradition of people looking in on people, making sure everybody's okay, being good company, that's a tradition that goes way back. Back to the time when folks painted rock art on stone faces by Lake Nemaska thousands of years ago. Maybe even further back than that.

Time passed, things changed.
Freddie's dad and the others who lived around there moved from their cabins and teepees into permanent houses clustered around the Hudson's Bay Trading Post. They built a good life.
Some things stayed the same. They still hunted, still looked in on each other, did some chores, had some tea and a smoke.
Some things changed. More white folks, white education, white problems. And in town everything was closer together than it

had been in the bush. In the bush, you had to walk everywhere. In town, you hardly had to walk at all.

Then Hudson's Bay closed their Nemaska trading post and the Province of Québec built the hydroelectric dam in the North. The engineers said the dam would change the course of water and Lake Nemaska would overflow the banks and submerge most of the town. Everything but the Hudson's Bay post, the burial grounds, and the steeple of the church. Their representative laid out charts and maps and told the elders that the people had to move.

So the folks of Nemaska scattered to the other Eeyou Istchee communities, mainly Mistissini and Waskaganish. They thought it would be a good time, thought that the other Eenou and Eeyou would welcome a few more people to their own communities and look in on them every now and again in a neighbourly sort of way.

That's not how it turned out to be.

For the people of Old Nemaska, it was a bad time. They were outsiders in the other communities and they were mistreated. Cheated, bullied, beaten, sometimes worse.

Freddie's dad went to Mistissini, and tried to fit in there. He didn't have it as bad as some of the others, but life in Mistissini sure wasn't great. Except that he found a girl he liked and married her and, soon after, in the hospital in Chibougamau, Freddie was born.

After seven years away, the news came that the people of Old Nemaska, who were having a bad time all around, were going to build a new Nemaska upriver from the old one, on Champion Lake.

Freddie's dad didn't have to think about it. He moved to new Nemaska and began looking in on the others there in a neighbourly sort of way.

It was good to be home.

FREDDIE WAPACHEE

Freddie grew up in the new town of Nemaska.

From time to time, his family went out on the land, where they hunted and ate traditional food. Rabbit, moose, goose, musk-rat, beaver, duck, bear, caribou, pheasant, grouse, ptarmigan, and more kinds of fish than you could list on a page.

The rest of the time they lived in town. Freddie had a life of routine. Woke up in the morning. Brushed his teeth and got dressed. Sat at the table and ate breakfast. Cereal and toast and jam and juice and eggs and bacon. Packed his bag and walked to school. Sat in class for a while, had a Rice Krispie square snack, went outside for recess. Sat in class some more and walked home for lunch. Sandwiches and soup and juice and cookies. Went back to school and sat in class for a while. Went outside again, kicked a ball around, in afternoon recess. Back inside for another hour of sitting in class. Went to the store after school for pop and chips. Walked home, hung out with friends, and watched TV. Ate dinner with the family. Pizza or goose with dumplings or fried chicken and poutine or whatever Freddie's mom cooked. Did his homework, then watched TV. Ate some popcorn or cheesies. Brushed his teeth and went to bed.

The next day, he did it all over again. That's town life for you.

After Freddie finished high school, first thing he did was take a week to do nothing.

Second thing he did was start training to be a police officer. After a week of basic training, he started working, and after a while he took some police courses, and then some more, and then, in '96, he took special constable training.

Mostly, he loved being a police officer. Mostly, Nemaska was a peaceful community and he liked the people. Best part of the job was to check in on folks in a neighbourly sort of way, just to see how they were doing. Run an errand if they needed it. Maybe even help someone change a tire. Usually they were happy to see him.

Worst part of the job was Freddie being too big to do some parts of the job. Sometimes a police officer had to be agile. Move quickly. Sometimes he had to run after someone or climb over something. That duty belt—fifteen pounds strapped to his waist—was a heavy thing and so was the bulletproof vest that all cops had to wear. Freddie was already a big guy. Moving quickly was hard to do. Strap on all that gear yet—and being agile was almost impossible.

After Freddie had been a police officer for a year, he married a girl from Waskaganish who already had a five-year old boy. Wasn't quite enough noise for them, so they had three more kids. Good kids, all four of them. Made him smile just to think about them.

It was a good life, all around.

Time passed, things changed.

In December of 2011, Freddie and his wife left the kids with family and drove to Ottawa to do some Christmas shopping. On the way back, their SUV heavy with gifts for the kids and big-box groceries, the windshield began to get blurry.

Not much of a surprise. You have to expect flurries in December.

Freddie turned on the wipers—but they didn't clear anything. Windshield was still blurry. And his wife was looking at him funny for turning them on. Like she didn't know what to make of it. The weather was fine, she said, the day was clear. There were no flurries.

What was not clear, what was as blurry as driving through a storm, was Freddie's vision.

Freddie reached for his face—maybe he had forgotten his driving glasses. But no, there they sat, on his nose like always.

He asked his wife for her glasses. They were a different prescription than his and they helped. Freddie wasn't sure he could pull off the look of ladies' glasses with bling on the rims, but at least he could see a little better and drive the rest of the way home.

The next day Freddie headed to the clinic.

They ran pretty much every medical test he had ever heard of and a few he hadn't. They pricked him with needles and listened to his heart and looked in his eyes. They had him stand on a scale and pee into cups. They poked and prodded, and they smeared his blood on a strip of paper and stuck it into a machine.

The machine said his blood sugar level was 20. When the clinic people saw that number, they pushed a fat needle into his arm, hooked him up to an IV, and pumped two full bags of fluid into him to bring the levels down to below 7.

No question at all. Freddie had type 2 diabetes.

Nemaska was a peaceful sort of place. When crime happened there, it usually had something to do with alcohol or drugs, with things people did when they were addicted. When they needed a little more of something and couldn't think on anything else. Made bad decisions. It was like that in small towns across Canada, anywhere unemployment was high and people got bored and frustrated.

Freddie worked in narcotics prevention. His job was to persuade folks that cocaine and heroin weren't worth it in the long run. He worked with kids in school before they even tried the stuff, and he taught them, with a big bear mascot, that substance abuse wasn't cool.

Not an easy job.

Usually, folks who were addicted wanted not to be addicted. Sometimes they were a little embarrassed about the drugs and scared to talk about what was going on at home. If someone like Freddie—a big guy in a uniform who carried a stick and looked a bit intimidating—approached them the wrong way, they just got more afraid. Then the addiction could get even worse and bad decisions could happen. But if he approached them another way, with understanding and trust, with being neighbourly and helpful and not punitive nor judgmental, then those same folks might ask him about treatment to recover from addiction. Or about how to keep their kids from trying drugs in the first place. Sometimes they didn't listen. Sometimes they did.

It wasn't so different from winter in the bush, from someone checking in to see did the old people have enough chopped wood for the day and did you have time for a cup of tea. But it wasn't easy.

As far as Freddie knew, there was no diabetes in his family. Other Cree had it. It was around the rez. That's about as much as he knew about it.

He drove home from the clinic, loaded his internet browser, and began to read about it. At first it was confusing. So many numbers, so much data. But he kept at it and after a week of reading, he mostly understood the disease. Then he began to read about the pills he was supposed to take. No way a narcotics prevention specialist like him was going to take pills he didn't understand. After a few more days of reading, he understood them too.

And what he also understood was that the Cree people used to move more than they do now. Living in the bush meant moving most of the time every single day. It was what the body wanted to do.

Another thing he understood was that diabetes was different for everyone. There were some people with diabetes who were skinnier than starving dogs at the end of winter. And there were some really big people who had no diabetes or high blood sugar or health problems at all.

But Freddie's diabetes had something to do with habits. Habits that had always felt like regular small town routine. A whole lot of sitting still, of driving everywhere, of eating more food than his body could use. Some of his habits began to look less like small town routine and a little more like the addiction-related habits of folks he worked with.

He was a narcotics-prevention specialist. Shouldn't have habits like those. As painful as it sounded, he was going to have to start to move.

Freddie had a treadmill at home. He began walking on it slowly for twenty minutes a day. It was exhausting. Sweat ran off him like rain until the treadmill belt was soaked. Every single muscle in his body ached.

Until, after a while, it wasn't so bad.

He headed outdoors then, to do his walking on the boardwalk at the outskirts of town. Just being there—sucking back the fresh air, gazing over the narrows, watching ducks paddle around, especially that one wounded duck that stayed year-round in the hot-spring culvert water, the duck that needed the kind of shelter you could get in Nemaska—all of it cleared the head.

Freddie began jogging a bit.

And then running.

With every new change, his muscles burned until he thought he couldn't take it. And then they got used to it.

The food habits were harder to break. Freddie cut down on pop and juice and began to drink water instead. He ate smaller portions at meals and stopped eating sweets altogether. Began to eat more of what his grandparents had eaten, more traditional food, and less of the store-bought kind.

And then the cravings came. Years ago, he had quit smoking, so he knew a thing or two about cravings. About habits that just would not give up. But this, this was something else. Freddie's stomach began to do battle with his brain. Bellowed at him for more food, for bigger meals and more snacks and a whole lot more sugar. His kids were eating as they always had, his stomach grumbled, why couldn't he? His stomach bellowed at him for eight whole months.

And then it gave up.

His stomach got used to the new habits, to smaller portions and less junk. It shrank. It shrank so much that when he ate a big meal, the sort he would have eaten before, he would vomit. Shrank so much that Freddie shrank too. Until about a hundred and twenty pounds were gone. A full third of him that wasn't there anymore.

He could move more easily now. He could run or jump over stuff at work when he had to, even with the duty belt on. He slept like a hibernating bear. He felt so much better. Looking back he saw that he had felt poorly for years without even knowing it.

Freddie is still a police officer in Nemaska. When he's on duty, he talks about narcotics prevention. When he's off duty, he talks about diabetes prevention. At tournaments, fitness challenges, feasts, any event where the Cree come together. If you see him, go over and say hello. Tell him about your day. Maybe he'll give you a free blood sugar test, just for fun. Maybe he'll tell you about all the walleye he and his kids caught this week when they were out fishing. Or about the elder on the corner who needs an extra hand. Or about teaching his kids to hunt at Old Nemaska Days when they all head back to the town that didn't flood after all, no matter what the engineers had said. The water levels are not what they once were, and the fish have changed their migratory patterns, but the old town is still there.

Some things have to change, and people will have to work to accept them. Some things should go back to the ways they used to be done. And some things ought to stay the same, just as they are. Neighbourliness, checking in on the people in your community who need a hand, those are things that should stay the same.

Epilogue

In 2018, ROSE SWALLOW retired from her work on the Chisasibi diabetes portfolio. She has six wonderful grandchildren who keep her very busy. She still loves spending time by herself and time on the land and looks forward to more of both. Her diabetes continues to be under control.

MAGGIE HAPPYJACK and SIMON ETAPP can often be seen at various sporting events and activities cheering on their grandkids. Simon works as Assistant Rehab Practitioner at (and driver for) the Waswanipi Multi-Service Day Centre. In January 2019, he had coronary bypass surgery and has recovered nicely. Maggie continues to work as Executive Secretary at CBHSSJB in Waswanipi. She's looking forward to retirement when she can spend more time at their bush camp. For both, the diabetes is under control.

ANNETTE SPENCER wanted to get back into hockey, but equipment proved too expensive in remote Whapmagoostui so she and her husband walk a great deal instead. She works two jobs and they are trying to give their kids an education that includes both college and traditional knowledge. They still spend as much time as they can at their bush camp—and they still take their TV with them. (The camp now has a permanent satellite dish.) Annette's diabetes was well-controlled until recently when she developed a liver condition for which she takes meds that affect her blood sugar. Annette and her husband are gradually figuring out a healthy family life under these new circumstances.

In addition to his job at the clinic, VARLEY MIANSCUM runs a thriving convenience store out of his basement. His diabetes remains the same, neither better nor worse. His father has passed away. At time of writing, Oujé-Bougoumou still had no Thai, Mexican, Chinese, Italian or fine dining restaurants. In fact, other than the Lodge diner (closed on weekends) and a canteen at the arena (also often closed), it had no restaurants at all.

SANDRA JUDITH BULLUCK continues to be highly involved in her community and to spend as much time as she can with her grandchildren. Since retiring and returning to a traditional diet, her diabetes has been under control. She hopes to go off all diabetes medication soon.

For a while, MARY NIQUANICAPPO lived in Montréal where she could walk easily and where she had a regular doctor. As a result, she was able to bring her diabetes under control, go off of insulin altogether, and lose 80 lbs. Now she's in Whapmagoostui again, where walking is not so easy, doctors not so regular, and diabetes control quite a bit more challenging. Thus far, though, she has managed and her blood sugar levels have been steady. Mary works two jobs, lives in her own home with her son (her grandmother has passed away), receives good support from the community and school, and is happy.

VICTOR GILPIN gets creative about staying fit. Recently, he cycled 60 km, ran a few half-marathons, tried out roller-blading, swimming, and hockey, and crossed a frozen 1.5 km-wide river, snow to his hips, without snowshoes, sinking every step of the way. When he's in the bush (which is as often as possible) he uses the snowmobile to haul wood, but does everything else (hunting, checking snares, and so forth) on foot. When he's in town, first thing, every morning, he's in the Eastmain gym, working out. The Residential School vegetable legacy continues: if he tastes certain vegetables, no matter how faintly, he is immediately nauseous. He sometimes does talks or presentations about living with diabetes. His diabetes is under control, his health is excellent, and he takes no medication.

Not long ago, KIMBERLY COON had a stroke affecting the left side of her body and making it difficult to walk. Since then, managing diabetes has been a struggle and she is trying to find a med regime that works under these new conditions. Her daughter left college temporarily to move home (along with her seven-year old daughter) and help out. Kim's continued work with Al-Anon is meaningful and provides her with skills helpful for diabetes management and for keeping a positive outlook. Her volunteer work for National Addictions Awareness is still a big part of her life.

JAMES JONAH has lived with diabetes for twenty years. He continues both to be thankful for the help he has received from Western doctors and to ask why Cree traditional medicines and expertise aren't being used more, especially since their track record is proven and since so many people are suffering. The community impact of people dying from diabetes or living with major diabetes complications is a significant source of stress and reminds him of how diabetes might yet affect him. Sometimes his motivation for diabetes control slides away for a while, but he makes a point of getting back on track quickly. James still works at the Waskaganish school.

MARTHA SHESHAMUSH lives with her diabetes under control. She takes no meds, has lost weight, and is happy to be smaller. As often as she can, she stays in the bush where stress quickly rolls away and where daily life demands that she keep moving. She still loves her work in Social Services where she supports people who are struggling with and recovering from addictions.

Since 2013, EMILY WESLEY has been the Public Health and Wellness Coordinator in Oujé-Bougoumou. She and her husband have four sons who keep them very busy. Her blood sugar levels are stable, her diabetes is under control, and she is happy.

LEONARD HOUSE continues to live in Chisasibi with diabetes as part of his life. Sometimes he wonders about how his health might be improved and hopes for a way out of his diabetes.

In December of 2020, CHRISTOPHER MERRIMAN turned 81. Once or twice a year, he heads back to Stratford-upon-Avon in England to check in with his family but he is always happy to return to Eastmain where he still works full time with the local Cree Nation as environment and land registry administrator. His neighbours keep him supplied with wild meat and blueberry pies. Thanks to Skype, he regularly connects with his grandkids (who call him Grampy). His health is good and his diabetes is under control.

Health, for JENNIFER SUSAN ANNISTIN, continues to be a rollicking adventure. In recent years, she's had a complete hysterectomy, an appendectomy, a months-long bout of shingles, and a surgery to remove four polyps from her colon—but her cancer is still in full remission and her diabetes continues to improve. She is stronger than ever and grateful for her rich life. From time to time she fosters children in her home.

Not long ago, RAQUEL EMMELINE WELSCH had a significant medication shift that did her a world of good. Her blood sugar levels are generally low and steady, and her health is excellent, especially for someone who has had diabetes for over forty years. On these new meds, she has lost over 20 pounds and with less weight to carry, finds it much easier to exercise. She still works full time but is looking forward to retirement in a couple of years, when she and her husband plan to move off-territory to the retirement house they've recently purchased.

JACK OTTER lives with his son in Waswanipi where he is both the Suicide Prevention officer of Waswanipi and the President of Dialogue for Life, a wellbeing and suicide prevention organization for Indigenous people of Québec. Despite some continued medical challenges (including bile duct cancer), Jack hunts in the bush—with one leg and no wheelchair—as often as he can. He takes Waswanipi youth with him, teaches them the Cree way of life on the land, and shows by example that giving up is never an option. Jack and his son spend as much time together as they possibly can.

LILLIAN MARTINHUNTER still works in Chisasibi with Youth Protection. After a five-year remission, her cancer returned, but she has now finished treatment and her health is on the mend again. She eats very carefully in order to control her sugar levels and, consequently, her need for medication has decreased significantly; she takes a fraction of the insulin she once took.

CAROLINE NEEPOSH passed away from cancer of the liver in the fall of 2018.

JONATHAN LINTON plays less hockey than he once did, and has taken up snowmobile racing. He's won some races—and others have left him with broken wrists, a concussion, and the like. He runs a year-around traditional camp for men with diabetes in which his clients learn to understand and control their diabetes and to reconnect with the land. Jonathan's own diabetes is under control and his health is good. Since telling his story in *The Sweet Bloods of Eeyou Istchee*, he has successfully hunted quite a few moose.

ANJA DIAMOND's health continues gradually to improve. She had a second surgery to treat the hernia, it brought some relief, and consequently she's been able to be more active—which is a good thing because her daughter, born in 2018, is full of energy and Anja often has to run after her. She takes her insulin and medications regularly, eats carefully, and feels much better than she once did. She has also signed up for gastric bypass surgery and is now undergoing the extensive training and preparation necessary for that life-altering procedure.

ANGELA ETAPP, who was once told by a doctor that she had 15-20 years to live, continues to be well and healthy, diabetes under control, long past that 20-year anniversary. She's the Coordinator of Administrative Services at the Waskaganish clinic. She makes a point of teaching her three teenaged kids about diabetes and encourages them to be as active as possible. In return, they keep her very busy.

JOEY BLACKSMITH passed away from diabetes-related complications in June of 2018.

COCO SIMONE CHANELLE continues to live in her community, diabetes under control. Her work travel schedule made strict diet control difficult, so Coco now travels with all of her food—snacks and meals carefully planned—so that there's no need for grocery-shopping or restaurant meals on the road. She walks regularly and she has a regular stretching regime to keep joints and muscles supple. She enjoys good relationships with her kids and grandkids, and she's out on the land, hunting and filling her freezer with small game, as often as her schedule allows.

FREDDIE WAPACHEE and his family moved to Waskaganish where Freddie is now the Lieutenant of the new Eeyou Eenou Police Detachment there. The move has been a positive one and they are settling well into community life. They have five grandkids and enjoy them a great deal. Reconciliation between Nemaska and other Eeyou Istchee communities has made significant headway and people on all sides continue to work at it. Freddie still enjoys good health. He eats carefully, exercises regularly, and checks in with his diabetes specialists. His meds have been reduced several times and he is off of insulin altogether.

We were unable to reach ELIZABETH BELL TAYLER or JENNIFER GLORIA LOWPEZ without compromising their confidentiality and therefore have nothing to report.

Glossary

An ADDICTION ENABLER is someone who tries to help fix another person's addiction, but who unintentionally makes it easier for the person to remain addicted. For instance, the enabler might try to preserve the addict's good reputation through a difficult time and cover up the addiction by making excuses for the addict, by calling in sick for her/him, or by cleaning up after her/him. Alternately, the enabler might organize her or his own life to prevent the addict's temper flareups or s/he might take the blame for the addict's harmful behaviour.

AL-ANON (which is not the same as Alcoholics Anonymous) is a group that provides support to friends and families of addicts in Eeyou Istchee and all around the world. In Mistissini, for example, the Al-Anon group meets on Tuesday evenings at 7 PM upstairs at the Mamou-Wechidodow Building on Amisk Street, and Ala-Teen meetings, for youth affected by people with addictions, are on Mondays at 3:30 PM at the Reception Centre, 282 Main Street. All of the meetings are open to the public. (These dates and addresses are current at time of writing.) The Al-Anon website is www.al-anon. org. See *Alcoholics Anonymous*.

ALCOHOLICS ANONYMOUS, or AA, is an international group that supports alcoholics in Eeyou Istchee and around the world as they try to become and stay sober. (In Mistissini, for instance, the AA group meets on Tuesday evenings at 7 PM downstairs at the Mamou-Wechidodow Building on Amisk Street.) AA is run mostly by people who are themselves recovering alcoholics. Because alcohols can be high in sugar (even if they don't taste sweet), people with diabetes sometimes choose to stop drinking alcohol altogether, and go to a support organization like AA for help in avoiding alcohol. The AA website is www.aa.org. See *Al-Anon.*

ASSIMILATION is one of those words that has more than one meaning. In this book, it refers to a dominant culture causing or forcing another culture to conform to its customs and attitudes and values, but at the same time limiting the assimilated culture's access to the benefits and privileges of the dominant culture. An assimilated culture is not likely to rise up and revolt against the dominant culture. Assimilation was and continues to be a tool used by colonizers in Canada: the First Nations were/are under enormous pressure to leave behind First Nations cultural ways and adopt the values and attitudes and customs of the dominant colonizing culture. See *colonization.*

BLOOD GLUCOSE is the fuel that we take from food and that gives energy to our bodies. In a person without diabetes, the fuel (glucose) goes from the blood to the organs that need it (with the assistance of insulin). In a person with diabetes, however, the fuel can't get to the organs, stays in the blood, and causes problems. See *diabetes, insulin.*

BLOOD SUGAR is another term for blood glucose. See *blood glucose.*

CARBOHYDRATES (Carbs) are one of the main sources of blood glucose fuel in our food. Carbs are found in many foods including those made of flour (bread, bannock, pasta) or fruit, in some alcohols, in potatoes, in any kind of desserts and sweets, and more. Because eating carbs can make a person's blood glucose increase quickly and dramatically, people with diabetes have to control very carefully how many carbs they eat and how often.

COLONIZATION is a method through which one country (or territory) takes over another country (or territory) in order to establish a colony. It involves taking control of the new land by using (and sometimes using up) its resources to make the colonizer stronger and richer and by sending people to occupy and govern the new country. Sometimes the occupiers use assimilation as a colonizing tool. The countries of France and England colonized the Indigenous lands and people of Canada. The process of colonization continues in Canada today. See *assimilation*.

C-SECTION is a short way of saying Caesarean Section. It is the surgery used when the baby is not born through the vagina but is instead born surgically and is cut out of the mother's uterus or womb. The name comes from the story that Julius Caesar (an ancient Roman military general and writer) was born in this way.

CURE is when a body recovers completely and permanently from an illness and has no remaining signs and symptoms of the illness. See *remission*.

DIABETES, or diabetes mellitus, is a group of diseases that affect the way a body processes blood sugar or blood glucose. Normally, the pancreas produces a hormone called insulin which controls the ways a body uses (or metabolizes) the fuel (glucose) we take in through eating. In a person with diabetes, however, either the pancreas can't produce insulin or the body can't use insulin properly, and the glucose can't get into the organs where it is needed. It stays in the blood instead and that person's blood glucose (or blood sugar) rises. A simple blood test shows if glucose is not being used properly: the blood glucose level will be too high, a condition called hyperglycemia. It is the main sign that a person has diabetes. (If someone's blood glucose level is too low, that person has hypoglycemia.) There are three types of diabetes: gestational diabetes affecting pregnant women and usually disappearing once the baby is born; type 1, in which the insulin-producing cells in the pancreas are destroyed as part of an autoimmune disorder; and type 2, in which the insulin-producing cells might be there, but either they don't produce the necessary insulin or the body resists what insulin they do produce. At time of writing, there is no guaranteed cure for type 1 or type 2 diabetes. Most of the diabetes in Eeyou Istchee is gestational or type 2 diabetes.

Diabetes can bring on heart disease, kidney failure, glaucoma and eventually blindness, chronic vaginal yeast infections, significantly reduced immune response and healing, anxiety, confusion, seizures, comas, nausea, abdominal pain, stroke, and more. See *blood sugar, cure, insulin, insulin resistance, pancreas, remission.*

DIALYSIS has more than one meaning, but in this book it refers to hemodialysis, a process whereby a machine does the work that a healthy kidney does naturally. Healthy kidneys clean the blood, regulate water and mineral levels, and add important substances. But if a person's kidneys are damaged and cannot clean the blood, toxins build up in the blood until the person enters a coma and eventually dies—unless that person regularly has dialysis. When someone is on dialysis, a machine is connected to the person's artery and vein (usually through tubes that run to an access point in the arm), the machine takes the blood from the artery, filters and purifies it, and then returns it to the vein. This process must be done every few days, so a person who needs dialysis can never be far from a dialysis machine.

GASTRIC BYPASS SURGERY is a radical surgery in which surgeons close off most of a person's stomach and fashion a small thumb-sized pouch in the upper part of the stomach. They attach the small intestine directly to the small pouch and the pouch becomes the person's new "stomach." After recovery, the person who has had the surgery can eat only tiny thumb-sized amounts of food for the rest of her or his life because that's all the pouch can hold. People who get gastric bypass surgery usually do it to help them lose weight but in rare cases people have the surgery done to help them manage diabetes.

HEMODIALYSIS is a type of dialysis. See *dialysis*.

INSULIN is a natural hormone, made in the pancreas. It has many jobs to do in a body—for instance, it affects memory and inflammation and healing—but its main job is to move sugar or glucose (fuel) from the blood into the cells and organs that use it for energy. Many people with diabetes inject a form of insulin that is very similar to their own natural insulin. A person might do this because his or her pancreas doesn't produce enough insulin or because the body can't use the insulin it does produce. See *diabetes, insulin resistance, pancreas.*

INSULIN RESISTANCE, or insulin resistance syndrome, is when someone's pancreas produces insulin, but the body tissues and cells are unable to use it efficiently. In response, the pancreas must produce more insulin than normal to get the glucose (fuel) into the cells—and eventually it can no longer keep up. Insulin resistance can happen as a result of aging, medications, lack of activity, obesity, trauma, malnutrition, genetic factors, and more. It is often associated with diabetes. See *insulin, pancreas.*

MISCARRIAGE is when the embryo comes out of the mother's body before it is a baby that can live on its own, Most often, miscarriage happens in the first three months of the pregnancy. A miscarriage is never intentional. (A pregnancy that is intentionally ended is called *abortion*.)

The PANCREAS is the large gland that produces insulin and helps with digestion. In a person with diabetes, the pancreas can burn out and produce less insulin than s/he needs. If that happens, doctors commonly recommend either pills that make the pancreas work harder or insulin that is injected directly into the body. Very rarely, a person with diabetes might get a pancreas transplant and that transplant might cure the diabetes—but it might not. (If, after a pancreas transplant, a person still has insulin resistance, then that person still has diabetes.) The pancreas lies behind the stomach. See *cure, insulin, insulin resistance.*

PRE-DIABETES often comes before type 2 diabetes. A person with pre-diabetes might not yet have all the symptoms of type 2 diabetes, but his or her blood glucose is already higher than it should be. Usually, pre-diabetes develops into type 2 diabetes. However, some people are able to stop this progression by making changes such as reducing their levels of stress, exercising more, or changing their diet.

REMISSION is when the signs and symptoms of a disease disappear for a period of time. When a person with diabetes goes into diabetes remission, her or his symptoms disappear and blood glucose returns to normal levels. Remission is less likely after someone has had diabetes for a long time. (Cancer is another group of diseases that sometimes goes into remission.) See *cure.*

TRADITIONAL FOODS in Eeyou Istchee are foods off the land, foods that the James Bay Cree have been eating for thousands of years. They include plants that have been gathered and animals that have been hunted or fished. Some Cree with type 2 diabetes who once ate a Western diet and then switched to a traditional diet have seen their diabetes symptoms reduce or even go away altogether.

YEAST INFECTION, or *candidiasis*, is a type of fungal infection that can grow on skin or under toenails, but most often it grows in parts of the body that produce mucous—like the throat or the vagina. Vaginal yeast infections, which can be caused by high blood glucose levels, can be a symptom of diabetes (the extra sugar in the blood throws off the natural vaginal yeast balance), but many women who get vaginal yeast infections do not have diabetes at all.

Conversations and Reflections on Diabetes and Colonization

WHEN James Bay Cree storytellers in this project talked to me about diabetes (or any illness), they often spoke of their physical health and wellness as being inseparable from spiritual health, from emotional health, from intellectual health, from community health, and from the health and wellness of the land. They used the word *miyupimaatisiiun,* loosely translated as being alive well in a way that encompasses all aspects of life (and native speakers of Cree emphasized the looseness of this translation). An illness like diabetes, then, was not only something having to do with the processing of blood glucose but was also intimately connected to the health and wellness of the other aspects of life.

Given that connection, it's no surprise that many storytellers mentioned to me that diabetes was virtually unheard of in Eeyou Istchee before the coming of the Europeans, before colonization. In those years, symptoms resembling diabetes symptoms appeared rarely, and, when they did, they could usually be treated with traditional medicines before they became a disease. Now, however, as this storybook demonstrates, the picture of diabetes on Eeyou Istchee is a different one altogether and diabetes prevalence is especially high. And Eeyou Istchee is not alone: Kevin Patterson, in his article "Diseases of Affluence,"[1] notes a similar pattern of high diabetes prevalence among other colonized Indigenous groups in Canada, United States, Australia, New Zealand, Marquesa Islands, Polynesia, Hawaii, Cook Islands, Tahiti, and a long list of other colonized locations around the world.

This pattern is important for two reasons. First, it suggests that the idea, often flippantly tossed into conversation, that type 2 diabetes is simply the consequence of bad choices (for instance, of eating too much or exercising too little) is far from accurate: a true picture is something more complex. Second, it reveals that, as people with diabetes and their various medical practitioners work to address the disease in Eeyou Istchee, part of what they are addressing is, in fact, the effects of a history of colonization.

During the process of collecting the stories gathered here and trying to understand diabetes in Eeyou Istchee, I had dozens of conversations in and around the subject of diabetes. They often turned towards specific aspects of colonization—aspects such as the long-term impact and far-reaching consequences of residential schools. Indigenous children across Canada were forced or strong-armed to attend Indian boarding schools that were administered by various Christian churches in Canada and eventually funded by the federal department of Indian Affairs and Northern Development. The earliest missionary boarding schools were run by the Récollets near Québec City from 1620 ending in 1680, and, in the 1820s and 1830s, churches began (with government involvement) to establish boarding schools for Indigenous children again. But it was in the 1850s, with the implementation of the Act to Encourage the Gradual Civilization of the Indian Tribes in this Province (1857), that assimilation through education became official government policy, and in the 1870s, with the implementation of the Indian Act (1869,

1. Patterson, Kevin. "Diseases of Affluence." *Maisonneuve* 35 (2010): 34-41. Print.

1876), that residential schools were established across Canada and caused widespread disruption of Indigenous culture. In 1920—despite continued reports of mishandled school administration and of starvation and neglect and abuse of students, including an especially damning 1907 school-conditions medical report submitted by Indian Affairs' Chief Medical Inspector Peter Bryce—residential school attendance became mandatory for Indigenous children in Canada. (Some parents, however, found ways to hide their children away.)

The residential schools had been established in part to fulfill treaty obligations of providing Indigenous children with education they might use to access Euro-Canadian society, but it quickly became clear that they had another agenda altogether. They existed mainly to cut Indigenous children off from their own culture and to assimilate them into dominant Canadian culture. The first paragraph of the *Summary of the Final Report of the Truth and Reconciliation Commission of Canada* says this:

> For over a century, the central goals of Canada's Aboriginal policy were to eliminate Aboriginal governments; ignore Aboriginal rights, terminate the Treaties; and, through a process of assimilation, cause Aboriginal peoples to cease to exist as distinct legal, social, cultural, religious, and racial entities in Canada. The establishment and operation of residential schools were a central element of this policy, which can best be described as 'cultural genocide.'[2]

The last residential school closed in 1996, only twenty years ago, and so a sizable portion of the storytellers who participated in this project either attended residential school or grew up with parents who attended; in Eeyou Istchee, the long-term impact and far-reaching consequences of the schools are felt and experienced

2. Truth and Reconciliation Commission. "Introduction." *Honouring the Truth, Reconciling for the Future: Summary of the Final Report of the Truth and Reconciliation Commission of Canada.* Jun 2015.

every day. The stories of individual experiences in the schools vary widely, depending on the residential schools the storytellers were sent to and the years they attended and what they wanted to share for this collection, but, repeatedly, stories of residential school include examples of trauma.

When it comes to diabetes, I heard again and again, trauma matters a great deal. Storytellers spoke to me of the ways in which trauma had disrupted their spiritual health, intellectual health, emotional health, and physical health. And medical practitioners talked about trauma or prolonged stress destabilizing the levels of insulin, the main controlling hormone in diabetes, and of malnutrition (common in some of the residential schools) and trauma as factors affecting insulin resistance. What it comes down to is that people who have experienced trauma are more susceptible to diabetes.

Another aspect of colonization that came up frequently in conversation is radical change in exercise and food practices. In traditional life of the James Bay Cree before colonization, insulin and blood glucose were regulated naturally.[3] Life on the land was intensely athletic and people spent waking hours moving, hauling water to cook, hunting on foot over vast regions, butchering animals that could be very large and heavy, treating and stretching and sewing their hides, chopping wood for cooking and staying warm, setting up and dismantling shelters and teepees in order to relocate to the next camp, and so forth. Further, the diet centred upon wild game, it included little in the way of sugar or flour, and it had built-in portion control because food had to last until the next hunt. Cree storytellers talked about this kind of life being inevitably healthier in part because of the intimate connection it nurtures with the land, and doctors and nurses and nutritionists pointed out the impact that exercise and a wild game diet have on the production of insulin and blood glucose levels in the body.

3. *Sweet Blood: Live Well with Diabetes.* Cree Board of Health and Social Services of James Bay (CBHSSJB). Dir. Shirley Cheechoo. 2009. DVD.

Of course, these traditions and ways of life never stopped being practised. They are still a vital part of everyday Eeyou Istchee life. But the ways they were (and continue to be) disrupted was something many people spoke of during the collecting of stories in this book. Storytellers talked about colonizers building trading posts and then airstrips and then roads that came up from the South. They talked of Indian Affairs pushing for the Eeyou and Eenou to leave behind nomadic ways and cluster in permanent settlements around the trading posts. (Some people stayed on the land year-round, but most moved into permanent settlements in and around the 1960s, still practising traditional hunting ways and going into the bush every year, but for shorter periods of time than they once had.) And they talked of roads from the South leading to the import of motorized vehicles so that, gradually, the people began using snowmobiles and all-terrain vehicles and trucks for travel, and they used the traditional methods of travel by dogsled or snowshoe or on foot less often than before. The James Bay Cree exercised altogether much less than they once had.

The ways of eating changed in Eeyou Istchee as well. Storytellers gave example after example of their traditional game diet with its natural protection against diabetes meeting formidable opposition in the residential schools. The schools forced upon them other ways of eating instead, ways that seemed alien to them, ways that were sometimes abusive, ways that were occasionally nutritious but were just as likely to starve them or make them quite sick, and ways that relied upon foods not traditionally available in Eeyou Istchee. Meanwhile, outside the schools, transport trucks, rolling up on new roads from the South, hauled boxes and boxes and boxes of processed foods to be sold in stores. The processed foods provided food options other than the traditional game diet, storytellers noted, but where wild game had given natural diabetes resistance, many of the processed foods stacked in tidy boxes on grocery store shelves were loaded with starches and other ingredients that raised blood glucose and made diabetes onset much more likely.

In an especially cruel coincidence, in the 1980s processed foods themselves changed in ways that made them even more unhealthy. Many of the packaged foods on the Canadian store shelves were actually American products, and, in United States, the Reagan administration introduced sugar quotas. These quotas prompted American food companies to use high-fructose corn syrup instead of sugar to sweeten packaged foods. In addition, the same administration, wanting fewer food industry regulations, allowed companies to use ingredients like aspartame that had never been allowed in food before. It didn't take long for high-fructose corn syrup and aspartame (and other ingredients) to be widely used in processed foods and to make their way onto shelves in Eeyou Istchee. But many years later, these very ingredients came under suspicion: at first, they had been hailed as healthy and safe, but now they were turning out to be unhealthy and unsafe after all, and especially for people with diabetes.[4]

Some of the older storytellers mentioned also the role played by the arrival of televisions and magazines in Eeyou Istchee in the late 1970s and 1980s, an arrival made possible by the new roads

4. In 2013, an article published in *Global Public Health* looked at statistics from 43 countries and found that countries commonly using high-fructose corn syrup as a sweetener in packaged foods had a 20% higher rate of diabetes than countries that didn't commonly use it. As for aspartame, an animal study suggested that it decreases insulin sensitivity in mice and makes the body require more insulin than it otherwise would, and another study found that meals with aspartame affect human insulin levels in the same way that meals with sugar do. Other studies similarly suggest that earlier claims about the safety of aspartame for people with diabetes are unreliable.

Goran, MI, SJ Ulijaszek, EE Ventura. "High Fructose Corn Syrup and Diabetes Prevalence: A Global Perspective." *Global Public Health* 8.1 (2013): 55-64. Web. 16 Feb 2016.

Collison, Kate, Nadine J Makhoul, Marya Zaidi, Soad Saleh, Bernard Andres, and Angela Inglis. "Gender Dimorphism in Aspartame-Induced Impairment of Spatial Cognition and Insulin Sensitivity." *PloS One* 7.4 (2012): e31570. Web. 15 Feb 2016.

Ferland, Annie, Patrice Brassard, and Paul Poirier. "Is Aspartame Really Safer in Reducing the Risk of Hypoglycemia During Exercise in Patients With Type 2 Diabetes?" *Diabetes Care* 30.7 (July 2007): e59. Web. 27 Feb 2016.

Sharma, Arun, S. Amaranth, M. Thulasimani, S. Ramaswamy. "Artificial Sweeteners as a Sugar Substitute: Are They Really Safe?" *Indian Journal of Pharmacology* 48.3 (May/June 2016): 237-240. Web. 7 Oct 2016.

from the South. The televisions and magazines quickly immersed the communities in food marketing the likes of which had never existed in the North before. In another coincidence, food marketing itself was changing rapidly at that very point in history. Marion Nestle notes:

> The early 1980s also marked the advent of the "shareholder-value movement" on Wall Street. Stockholder demands for higher short-term returns on investments forced food companies to expand sales in a marketplace that already contained excessive calories. Food companies responded by seeking new sales and marketing opportunities. They encouraged formerly shunned practices that eventually changed social norms, such as frequent between-meal snacking . . . and serving larger portions. (41)[5]

With their traditional food patterns disrupted, many Eeyou and Eenou had taken packaged foods, stuffed with ingredients that caused blood glucose problems, into their post-residential school diet. Marketing also took its toll and average food portions grew in size as mealtimes and snacking became more frequent than the traditional diet had allowed. Food, the basic nutrition a human being cannot live without, had become a tool in colonization and assimilation.

One of the colonization events that most affected the James Bay Cree of Northern Québec was the James Bay Hydroelectric Project. Each storyteller who mentioned it, and many did, revealed more ways it had caused distress for the Eeyou and Eenou. In the mid-1970s, the Province of Québec and Hydro-Québec initiated a hydroelectric project. It was going to be one of the biggest in the world and would generate electricity they could sell, mostly to United States. The project itself, they decided, would be located in

---

5. Nestle, Marion. "Eating Made Simple." *Scientific American: The Science of Food: Special Collector's Edition* Summer 2015: 39-45. Print.

the North on traditional Cree and Inuit land—but they started the project without once consulting the Cree or Inuit.

Indigenous land and livelihoods had already been affected by forestry and mining in northern Québec, but the James Bay Hydroelectric Project was on another scale altogether. The construction of it involved massive upheaval of the northern landscape. Some storytellers described dams being constructed, others spoke of the diversion of nine rivers, others mentioned the flooding of 11,500 square kilometres of wilderness, others were frustrated by the impact on Cree lives when animal migration routes were altered or when fish became contaminated by mercury or when approximately 10,000 caribou were poisoned to death, and many recalled the turmoil and socially toxic aftermath that followed the relocation of two whole communities: the houses of Fort George had to be removed from their foundations, set on trucks and barges, and hauled 14 kilometres upriver to Chisasibi, and the town of Nemaska was left behind and eventually rebuilt in another area altogether. And then there was the James Bay Road. The dams couldn't be built without big construction machines, and, to get the machines to where they had to be, an entire highway, 620 kilometres long, had to be built up the eastern side of James Bay. With the highway came still more colonizers, still more processed foods, more exercise-avoidance machines, more disruption of food and water and livelihood, and much more stress.

The James Bay Cree, of course, did not take this incursion lightly. The ensuing legal battles, spearheaded by Billy Diamond from the Cree Nation of Waskaganish, tied up courts for years and resulted in the creation of the James Bay and Northern Québec Agreement in 1975. When, in the late 1980s, a second phase of the James Bay Hydroelectic Project began, Cree activists were ready. They headed to legislatures in United States and lobbied against purchasing electricity from the James Bay Project. They kept on lobbying until New York Power Authority eventually cancelled its contract with Hydro-Québec and that phase of the James Bay Project was put on hold for lack of a market.[6]

Storytellers pointed out that the James Bay Northern Québec Agreement (signed by the Grand Council of the Crees, the Northern Québec Inuit Association, Hydro-Québec, and the governments of Canada and Québec) did begin to address some of the ways in which the James Bay Cree had been mistreated through colonization and by colonizers and by the Hydroelectric Project. But damage had been done; after the dust had settled, it became clear to Cree Board of Health and Social Services of James Bay that the areas most affected by the James Bay Hydroelectric Project were the same areas that had the highest percentages of people with diabetes.

One of the purposes of this storybook is to share some of the many ways that storytellers in Eeyou Istchee live with and think about diabetes, and to encourage others to talk more about it. For many Eeyou and Eenou, diabetes and its complicated history and context affect all aspects of life—there's still plenty to talk about. We've hardly scratched the surface.

Ruth DyckFehderau

6. "James Bay Project." *The Canadian Encyclopedia.* Historica Canada, 2016. Web. 31 Mar 2016.

Acknowledgements

WRITING is a collaborative art and I could not have completed this storybook alone. My thanks go, above all, to each storyteller herein who worked patiently with me. Thanks also to Paul Linton, the CBHSSJB Assistant Director of Public Health for Chishaayiyuu (adults). His unwavering support, guidance, wisdom, and trust in the years it took me to finish, all without once being intrusive or heavy-handed, made this project a pleasure to work on, something to look forward to each day. The Community Health Representatives (CHRs) of Cree Board of Health and Social Services of James Bay selected storytellers for this project, arranged appointments, and provided other support during my trips to the communities: Amy Dick and Jean Masty of Whapmagoostui, Rose Iserhoff of Chisasibi, Laurie-Ann Georgekish of Wemindji, Ena Weapenicappo of Eastmain, Verna Jolly of Waskaganish, Bella Jolly of Nemaska, Diane Ottereyes of Waswanipi, Jennifer Pepabano of Oujé-Bougoumou, and Jonathan Linton of Mistissini. Additional community support came from Veronique Doutreloux in Nemaska, Martin Lewis in Oujé-Bougoumou, Monique Laliberté in Mistissini, Mina House in Chasasibi (who tracked down participants, explained local history, and provided excellent company and good humour between meetings), CBHSSJB drivers who transported me to and from airports, and cleaning staff who prepared transits. Gabriel Doutreloux drove me across Eeyou Istchee expanses and went far beyond what his company (Allô Taxi) was contracted to do. Catherine Godin, Hélène Porada, and Roberta Petawabano willingly shared their considerable diabetes expertise, and Dr. Rosy Khurano answered medical questions any time I asked them. Ron Shisheesh taught me about gun-shopping. Martha McKenzie and Victor Gilpin put extra time into explaining aspects of local and Indigenous history. Solomon Awashish, accomplished storyteller that he is, expertly answered dozens of questions about Cree history and culture, often in ways that left my gut sore from laughter. Catherine Gutwin helped sort out sentence-level writing problems along the way and Srilata Ravi edited my French. Norma Dunning read the manuscript and generously shared sharp, insightful, and much-needed commentary. Cameron Mosimann donated his time and skill to design the book cover. Peter Midgley of University of Alberta Press gave me invaluable advice, both in thinking through Indigenous storytelling and in book production, and Kelly Boon, Sarah Elash, and the folks at Houghton Boston patiently offered ample book production assistance. Manikarnika Kanjilal copyedited the second edition, and a number of visually impaired readers, who preferred not to be named but to whom I am forever grateful, made recommendations for accessible design. Jocelyn Brown, artist and copyeditor and accessible design consultant and content editor rolled into one remarkable person, carefully edited this manuscript with sharp eye and considerable finesse, and Alison Scott graciously proofread and polished and updated the design for the second edition. And finally, David DyckFehderau (known in Eeyou Istchee as "DuckFeathers"): Greater love hath no man than this, that he listen to a 280-page book being read aloud to him in its entirety—twice!!—and each time pass on support and astute critique. David also provided the cover photograph and helped with everything from flight bookings to hunting down storytellers on foot to book design to a thousand other things in between.

Ruth DyckFehderau teaches Creative Writing and English Literature at the University of Alberta for a few months of each year and the rest of the time she travels and writes. Her work has been published in literary journals and anthologies around the world, and she has received awards for writing, teaching, and activism. For two years, while writing this book, she lived in Eeyou Istchee. She is currently based in Edmonton, Alberta.

Coming Soon from
Cree Board of Health and Social Services of James Bay

Finding Our Way Home

Residential School Recovery Stories
of the James Bay Cree: Volume 1

Stories by James Bay Cree Storytellers
Written by Ruth DyckFehderau
Distributed by Wilfrid Laurier University Press

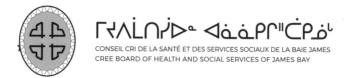

ᒥᔅᐱᓂᒡᐃᐧᐊᐣ ᐊᐧᐋᐱᒋᐦᑖᑲᓄᒡ

CONSEIL CRI DE LA SANTÉ ET DES SERVICES SOCIAUX DE LA BAIE JAMES
CREE BOARD OF HEALTH AND SOCIAL SERVICES OF JAMES BAY